Nesrine Souayeh
Azza Laaouini
Hajer Bettaieb

Model M4 and HCG ratio

Nesrine Souayeh
Azza Laaouini
Hajer Bettaieb

Model M4 and HCG ratio

Performance in predicting the outcome of pregnancies of undetermined location

ScienciaScripts

Imprint
Any brand names and product names mentioned in this book are subject to trademark, brand or patent protection and are trademarks or registered trademarks of their respective holders. The use of brand names, product names, common names, trade names, product descriptions etc. even without a particular marking in this work is in no way to be construed to mean that such names may be regarded as unrestricted in respect of trademark and brand protection legislation and could thus be used by anyone.

Cover image: www.ingimage.com

This book is a translation from the original published under ISBN 978-620-6-71441-5.

Publisher:
Sciencia Scripts
is a trademark of
Dodo Books Indian Ocean Ltd. and OmniScriptum S.R.L publishing group

120 High Road, East Finchley, London, N2 9ED, United Kingdom
Str. Armeneasca 28/1, office 1, Chisinau MD-2012, Republic of Moldova, Europe
Printed at: see last page
ISBN: 978-620-7-74518-0

TABLE OF CONTENTS

INTRODUCTION

Pregnancy with indeterminate location (GLI) is defined as the situation in which a pregnancy is objectified by a urine or blood test while endovaginal ultrasound (EEV) does not initially allow the location of the pregnancy to be specified (intrauterine or extrauterine) [1].

This is not a diagnosis, but rather an intermediate classification pending the final outcome, which may be favorable toward a viable or non-viable intrauterine pregnancy (IUP), or a failed GLI, or unfavorable toward a persistent GLI or ectopic pregnancy (EP). [2]. Consequently, follow-up with additional clinical and para-clinical examinations is then necessary before the location and/or viability of a pregnancy can be defined. [1].

The incidence of GLI is gradually increasing, and currently accounts for between 8% and 10% of consultations in gynecological emergencies. [3,4]. It thus continues to be a subject of concern and a source of anxiety for both patient and practitioner. [[5].

In 0.03% to 2.4% of cases, GLI progresses to a ruptured ectopic pregnancy (EP) requiring emergency surgical management and blood transfusion. [6,7].

In order to avoid repetitive ß -HCG assays and unnecessary hospital admissions, several biomarkers have been proposed to stratify the evolutive risk of GLI, the most widely used of which are serum progesterone and the HCG ratio. [2].

Based on these parameters, mathematical models have also been developed, such as the M4 model and, more recently, the M6 model. These models have the advantage of classifying certain patients in the low-risk group for ectopic pregnancy as early as the first consultation, with a better performance for the M6 model thanks to the integration of the initial progesterone level [8].

However, the guidelines of the various learned societies are heterogeneous with regard to the choice of biomarker to be used and the cut-offs to be considered for the different mathematical models. Moreover, no Tunisian study has evaluated the use of these methods in the triage of GLI, where access to emergency serum progesterone measurement remains very limited.

With this in mind, we conducted this study to assess the performance of the M4 model and the HCG ratio in risk stratification of pregnancies of undetermined location (GLI).

MATERIALS AND METHODS

1. Presentation of the study

1.1 Type of study

This was a single-center, retrospective, descriptive and analytical study of 384 cases of pregnancy with indeterminate localization (GLI).

1.2 Scope and location of the study

This study was carried out in the obstetrics and gynecology department of the Ben Arous regional hospital. This is a level IIB maternity hospital providing obstetrics, medical gynecology, gynecological surgery for benign pathologies and gynecological carcinological surgery to the southern suburbs of Tunis.

1.3. Study period

Our study was conducted over a period of 6 years and 4 months, from January 1, 2017 to April 30, 2023.

2. Study population

2.1. Inclusion criteria

We included patients who consulted our emergency department and had a positive ß -HCG assay on biology without obvious signs of ectopic pregnancy (EP) or intrauterine pregnancy (IUP) on ultrasound.

2.2 Non-inclusion criteria

We did not include in our study :

- Patients with an unstable hemodynamic state on admission.
- Patients with abnormalities on initial ultrasound: latero-uterine mass, pelvic effusion, doubt about an intrauterine gestational sac.

2.3 Exclusion criteria

We have excluded from our study :

- Patients whose GLI outcome was unknown.
- Patients diagnosed with EP or UGI within the first 48 hours of hospitalization.
- Patients who have not had a ß -HCG assay after 48 hours of the first assay.
- Patients who have progressed to persistent gestational trophoblastic disease.

2.4. Judging criteria

The primary endpoint was pregnancy outcome with indeterminate location defined as follows, according to the consensus nomenclature established by Barnhart et al in 2011 (Appendix 1):

1) GLI failure: if the serum ß -HCG level has dropped to 25 IU/L or less (negative assay).

2) Ectopic pregnancy: if an ectopic pregnancy was visible on endovaginal ultrasound (EEV) or at laparoscopy, and if ß -HCG levels were static (variation of less than 15% every 48 hours on three consecutive determinations).

3) Intrauterine pregnancy: if a gestational sac has been visualized on EEV with or without a yolk vesicle or heterogeneous tissue in the uterine cavity consistent with products of conception on aspiration.

4) Persistent GLI: if the ß -HCG level does not decrease spontaneously, or there is an abnormal increase or plateau (a variation of less than 15% over three consecutive measurements at 48-hour intervals), and the

endovaginal ultrasound (EEV) shows no intrauterine or extrauterine pregnancy.

3. Methods

3.1 Calculating sample size

To calculate the sample size required to obtain statistically significant results, we used the following formula:

$$\text{Ideal sample size} = \frac{(Score\ Z)^2 \times ecart\ type \times (1-ecart\ type)}{(marge\ d'erreur)^2}$$

With :

- Z score = 1.96 (representing the critical value associated with the desired 95% confidence level)
- 5% standard deviation
- Margin of error at 5%.

Sample size= ((1.96) 2x 0.5 x (0.5)) / 0.052 ≈ 384

3.2. Scores evaluated

3.2.1. HCG ratio

The HCG ratio is defined as the HCG level at 48 hours divided by the initial HCG dosage. To assess its relevance in GLI risk starification, we used the following cut-offs, referring to the most recent data in the literature (Appendix 2):

- A ratio of less than 0.87 (indicating a drop in HCG levels of at least 13% over 48 hours) is considered compatible with a final result of GLI failure.
- A ratio greater than 1.66 is likely to lead to a final result of intrauterine pregnancy (IUP).

- And a ratio between these two values is more indicative of an ectopic pregnancy or persistent GLI.

3.2.2. Model M4

Model M4 is a mathematical logistic regression model based on initial serum HCG dosage and HCG ratio as variables. For each patient, it calculates the probability of intrauterine pregnancy, EP and GLI failure. The patient is considered at high risk if the risk of EP was greater than or equal to 5% (Appendix 3).

3.2.3. Estimated actual expenditure

The cost of managing the patients included in our study was estimated by calculating the expenses incurred for additional tests (in particular ß-HCG assays and ultrasound scans), diagnostic procedures (uterine revisions, diagnostic laparoscopies), and the cost of the hospital stay required to reach the final diagnosis.

3.2.4. Estimated theoretical expenditure

For all patients, we estimated the theoretical cost of management by calculating the theoretical expenses with reference to the risk classification by the scores studied:

3.2.4.1. Estimated expenditure if triage by HCG ratio were applied

For all patients, we estimated the theoretical expenditure if we applied the algorithm below (Figure 1), inspired by the work of Bobdiwala et al (Appendix 2).

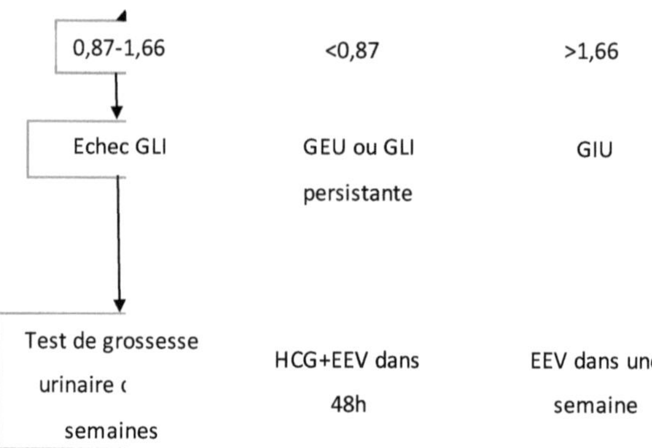

EEV: endovaginal pelvic ultrasound; GLI: pregnancy of undetermined location; GEU: extra uterine pregnancy; GIU: intra uterine pregnancy; HCG: human chorionic gonadotropin.

Figure 1HCG ratio triage and management algorithm for GLI

3.2.4.2. Estimated expenditure if sorting by the M4 model were applied

For all patients, we also estimated the theoretical expenditure if we applied the triage algorithm by the model M4 proposed by Bobdwila et al. (Figure 2) (Appendix 4).

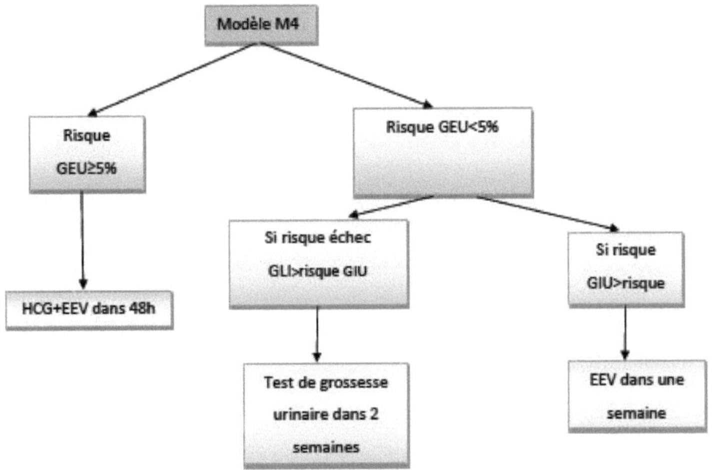

EEV: endovaginal pelvic ultrasound; GLI: pregnancy of undetermined location; GEU: extra uterine pregnancy; GIU: intra uterine pregnancy; HCG: human chorionic gonadotropin.

Figure 2Algorithm for sorting and handling GLI by the M4 model

3.2.5. Estimated savings

The expenditure saved was estimated by calculating the difference between the actual expenditure deployed to reach the final diagnosis and the "theoretical" expenditure that would have been deployed if the HCG ratio and the M4 model had been integrated.

3.3. Data collection

A pre-established data collection form was used for all patients (Appendix 5).

Data were collected from the medical records of patients who were hospitalized in the obstetrics gynecology department at Ben Arous regional hospital for GLI.

3.3.1. Medical history data

The questioning allowed us to specify:

- Age
- Geographical origin
- Civil status
- Medical and surgical history
- Gyneco-obstetrical history: gestiture, parity, mode of delivery, menarche, regularity and duration of menstrual cycle, date of last menstrual period (DDR) and duration of amenorrhea, notion of dysmenorrhea or dyspareunia, history (ATCD) of tubal plasty, endometriosis, infertility, EP or upper genital infection (UGI).
- Contraception
- Smoking
- Recourse to medically assisted procreation (MAP)
- And finally, the reason for consultation: metrorrhagia, pelvic pain, sympathetic signs of pregnancy, ...

3.3.2. Physical examination data

The physical examination revealed :

- Assess general condition, state of consciousness and mucocutaneous pallor
- Measure hemodynamic constants (blood pressure and pulse) and temperature

- Look for pelvic tenderness or discomfort and specify the site

- Look for the presence or absence of metrorrhagia, specify the opening of the uterine cervix, presence or absence of an adnexal mass or pain in the cul de sac (CDS) on vaginal touch and speculum examination.

3.3.3. Paraclinical data

3.3.3.1. Biological tests

For all patients, we specified the results of the following biological examinations:

- Initial and 48-hour ß-HCG assays

- Blood count

- Prothrombin rate (PT) and activated partial thromboplastin time (APTT)

We also recorded the number of ß-HCG assays required to reach the final diagnosis.

3.3.3.2. Pelvic ultrasound data

All patients included in our study underwent suprapubic and endovaginal pelvic ultrasonography. We reported the thickness of the endometrium, the appearance of the adnexa, the presence or absence of intraperitoneal effusion and its abundance.

We also recorded the number of pelvic ultrasounds required to reach the final diagnosis.

3.3.4. Care and maintenance

The management of GLI in the Ben Arous obstetrics and gynecology department follows a protocol drawn up within the department (Appendix 2).

For all patients, we reported the length of hospital stay and the diagnostic and therapeutic procedures performed.

3.4. Statistical analysis

Data were entered and analyzed using Statistical Package for Social Science (SPSS) version 26.

3.4.1. Descriptive study

We calculated absolute frequencies and relative frequencies (percentages) for categorical variables.

For quantitative variables, we calculated means, medians and standard deviations, and determined extreme values.

3.4.2. Analytical study

Patients were risk-stratified using the HCG ratio and the M4 model.

A second classification was made according to the selected diagnosis. According to the final diagnosis, our population was divided into three groups as follows:

- ➢ Group 1 (G1): Ectopic pregnancy (EP)
- ➢ Group 2 (G2): progressive intrauterine pregnancy (GIU)
- ➢ Group 3 (G3): non-progressive intrauterine pregnancy or failed pregnancy of undetermined location (GLI)

Comparisons of three means on independent series were carried out using Student's t-test for independent series and the non-parametric Kruskal walis test.

Percentage comparisons on independent series were carried out using Pearson's chi-square test, and in the event of significance in the chi-square test and non-validity of this test and comparison of 2 percentages, by Fisher's two-tailed exact test.

To identify independent factors, we used binary logistic regression, considering factors with a significance level (p) of less than 0.2.

The measure of association was the Odds Ratio (OR) and its 95% confidence interval [IC95%].

In all statistical tests, the significance level was set at 0.05.

4. Bibliographic research

The bibliographical search was based on :

- Search engines such as Pubmed, Google Scholar and science direct using keywords.
- Theses available in Tunisian medical schools and international theses available on the Internet.

We used the following keywords in accordance with MeSH guidelines: ectopic pregnancy, terminated pregnancy, mathematical model, HCG ratio, prognosis; to carry out targeted searches of scientific articles.

References have been written according to VANCOUVER's recommendations and arranged in the order in which they appear in the text.

5. Ethical considerations

As our study was retrospective, it had no impact on the quality of patient care. When processing the data, we respected the principles of anonymity and medical confidentiality. The results will be accessible to all researchers interested in this field.

6. Conflicts of interest

We declare no conflicts of interest.

RESULTS

1. Epidemiological characteristics of the study population

From January 1, 2017 to April 30, 2023, 30463 women were admitted to the obstetrics and gynecology department at Ben Arous Regional Hospital for obstetric and gynecological pathologies. Among these patients, 613 women had at least one pathological sign of early pregnancy, a frequency of 2.01%.

After excluding women with an unstable hemodynamic state on admission and/or abnormalities on initial ultrasound (n=195), we excluded 34 cases according to our exclusion criteria. We thus retained 384 patients with a positive ß-HCG assay on biology, with no obvious sign of extra-uterine pregnancy (EUP) or intra-uterine pregnancy (IUP) on ultrasound (Figure 3).

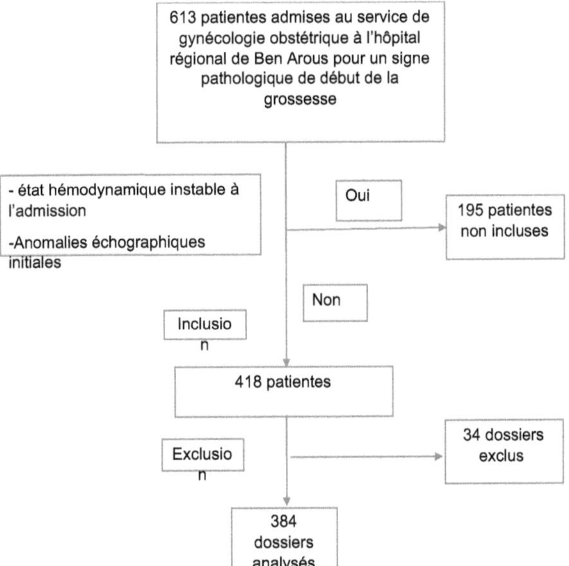

Figure 3Flow chart

1.1 Incidence and prevalence of pregnancy of undetermined location

Annual incidence was estimated at an average of 55 cases/year, representing a prevalence of 1.4% (Figure 4).

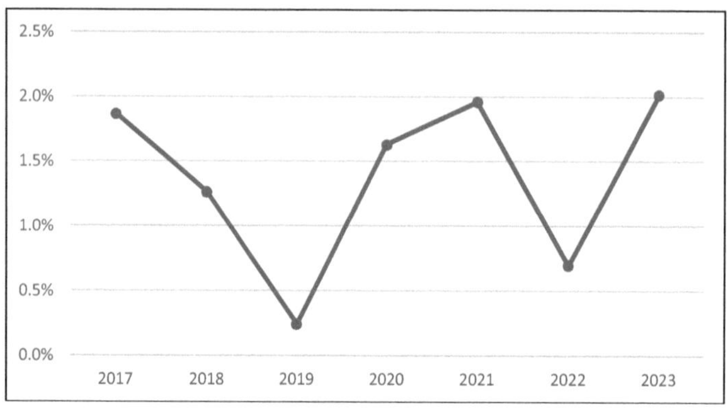

Figure 4Distribution of patients by annual incidence of pregnancies of undetermined location

According to the final diagnosis retained, our population was divided into three groups as follows (Figure 5):

> ➢ Group 1 (G1): 151 cases of EP (39%).

> ➢ Group 2 (G2): 61 cases of progressive intrauterine pregnancy (16%).

> ➢ Group 3 (G3): 172 cases of non-progressive intrauterine pregnancy or failed pregnancy of undetermined location (GLI), i.e. 45%.

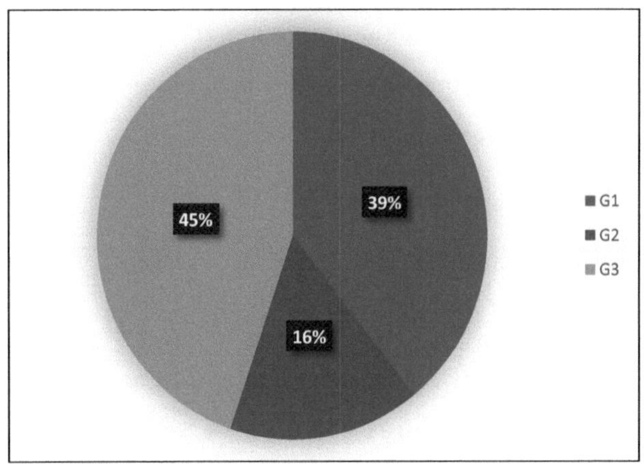

Figure 5Distribution of patients according to final diagnosis

1.2. Age

The mean age of our patients was 32.8±5.7 years, with extremes ranging from 18 to 46 years, and 34.4% of patients were over 35 years of age (n=132).

The figure below illustrates the distribution of patients by age (Figure 6).

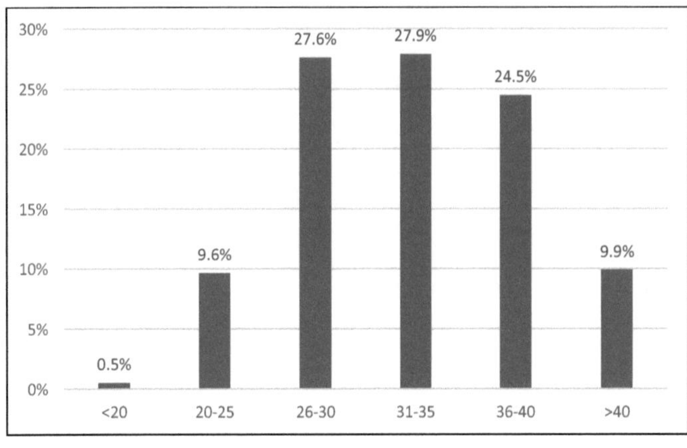

Figure 6Age distribution of patients

A comparative study of the three groups according to age showed that the age of patients in groups G1 and G3 was significantly higher than in group G2 (p=0.042) (Table I).

1.3 Gestité

The average gestational age of our patients was 3±1.8, with extremes ranging from 1 to 12.

Furthermore, there was no significant difference between the three groups in terms of gestia (p=0.317) (Table I).

1.4. Parity

The mean parity of our patients was 1.38±1.1, with extremes ranging from 0 to 5.

The parity of groups 1 and 3 was significantly higher than that of group 2 (p=0.008) (Table I).

Table IEpidemiological data for our study population

		Average	Standard deviation	Minimum	Maximum	P
Age	**G1**	33	5,2	22	46	0,042
	G2	31,1	5,9	19	45	
	G3	33,24	6,2	18	44	
	Total	32,81	5,8	18	46	
Gestité	**G1**	3	1,9	1	12	0,317
	G2	2,5	1,5	1	6	
	G3	3,2	1,8	1	12	
	Total	3	1,8	1	12	
Parity	**G1**	1,1	1,1	0	4	0,008
	G2	0,9	1,1	0	4	
	G3	1,4	1,2	0	5	
	Total	1,38	1,1	0	5	

G1: ectopic pregnancy; G2: progressive intrauterine pregnancy; G3: non-progressive intrauterine pregnancy or failed pregnancy of undetermined location (GLI)

1.5. Risk factors for ectopic pregnancy

1.5.1. Previous ectopic pregnancy

A history of ectopic pregnancy (EP) was found in 33 patients (8.6%). Comparison of the 3 groups showed a significantly higher rate of EP in group 1 (p=0.032) (Table II).

1.5.2. Previous caesarean section

One hundred and fourteen patients, or 29.7%, had at least one caesarean section. The average number of caesarean sections was 1.44±0.5, with extremes of 1 to 4.

Comparing the 3 groups for cesarean section history, there was no significant difference (p=0 .266) (Table II).

1.5.3. History of pelvic surgery

A history of pelvic surgery was found in 27 patients (7%), distributed as follows: Appendectomy in 17 women (7 cases by laparoscopic approach and 10 by Mac Burney approach), cystectomy in 8 women (6 cases by laparoscopic approach and 2 cases by laparotomy) and myomectomy in two cases, both approached by laparotomy (Table II).

For previous appendectomy, there was no significant difference between the 3 groups (P=0.406).

1.5.4. History of tubal plasty

A history of tubal plasty was found only in 7 patients (1.8%): 6 patients in group G1 (4%) and one patient in group G2 (1.6%). The difference between groups was statistically significant (p=0.008) (Table II).

1.5.5. History of infertility

A history of infertility was noted in 16 cases: 9 patients in group G1, 5 patients in group G2 and 2 patients in group G3.

Four patients with a history of infertility had conceived by ovulation inducer, one of whom required intrauterine insemination with the spouse's sperm.

For previous infertility, there was a significant difference, with a higher rate among patients in group G1 (p=0.028) (Table II).

1.5.6. History of upper genital infection

A history of upper genital infection (UGI) was noted in 6 cases (1.56%): 3 patients in group 1 (0.78%), one patient in group 2 (0.78%) and 2 patients in group 3 (0.52%). Although IGH was more frequent in group 1, the difference between the 3 groups was not significant (p=0.552) (Table II).

1.5.7. Contraception

Seventy-four patients (19.27%) had used contraception in the previous 3 months. The most common form of contraception was the microprogestogen pill, found in 41 patients (10.76%), followed by the intrauterine device (IUD) (n=15; 3.9%). The difference between groups in contraceptive type was not statistically significant.

1.5.8. Smoking

Our population included 43 patients who used tobacco (11.19%).

Although the smoking rate was higher in group 1, the difference with the other groups was not statistically significant (p=0.679) (Table II).

Table IISummary table of the main risk factors for ectopic pregnancy

		Mean± Standard deviation	Minimum	Maximum	P
Caesarean section history	G1	1,49±0,59	1	3	0,266
	G2	1,24±0,44	1	2	
	G3	1,48±0,6	1	4	
	Total	1,44±0,5	1	4	
		Workforce		Percentage (%)	P
History of EP	G1	17		11,3	0,032
	G2	8		13,1	
	G3	8		4,7	
	Total	33		8,6	
		Workforce		Percentage (%)	P
History of pelvic surgery	G1	10		6,6	0
	G2	2		3,3	,443
	G3	15		8,7	
	Total	27		7	
		Workforce		Percentage (%)	P
History of tubal plasty	G1	6		4	0,008
	G2	1		1,6	
	G3	0		0	
	Total	7		1,8	
		Workforce		Percentage (%)	P
History of infertility	G1	9		6	0,028
	G2	5		8,2	
	G3	2		1,2	
	Total	16		4,2	
		Workforce		Percentage (%)	P
IGH history	G1	3		0,78	0,552
	G2	1		0,26	
	G3	2		0,52	
	Total	6		1,56	
		Workforce		Percentage (%)	P
Smoking	G1	20		13 ,2	0,679
	G2	3		4,9	
	G3	20		11,6	
	Total	43		11,19	

G1: Ectopic pregnancy; G2: Progressive intrauterine pregnancy; G3: Non-progressive intrauterine pregnancy or failed pregnancy with undetermined location (GLI); Past history; EUS: Extrauterine pregnancy; IUD: Intrauterine device; IGH: Genital infection.

2. Clinical study

2.1. Functional signs

2.1.1. Duration of amenorrhea

The mean duration of amenorrhea was 6.37 weeks, ranging from 4 to 14.4 weeks.

Amenorrhea was significantly longer in group 3 (p<0.001) (Table III).

Table IIIDistribution of patients by group and amenorrhea duration

Duration	Average	Standard deviation	Minimum	Maximum	p
G1	6,24	1,50	4	13,6	<0,001
G2	5,49	1,21	4	8,6	
G3	6,79	1,99	4	14,4	
Total	6,37	1,75	4	14,4	

G1: ectopic pregnancy; G2: progressive intrauterine pregnancy; G3: non-progressive intrauterine pregnancy or failed pregnancy of undetermined location (GLI)

2.1.2. Pelvic pain

On admission, 295 patients (76.82%) presented with pelvic pain (figure 7).

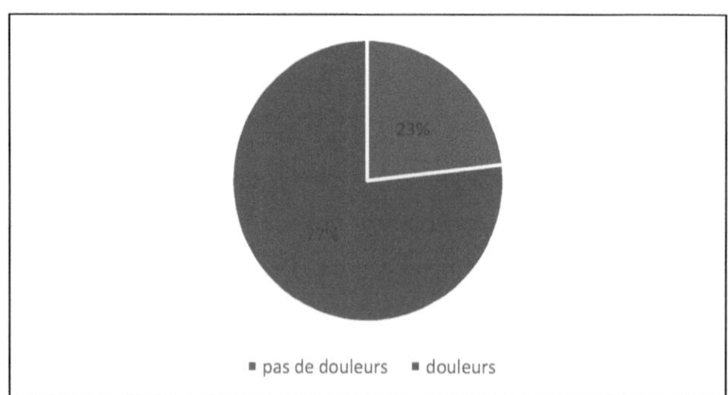

Figure 7Distribution of patients according to the presence or absence of pelvic pain

Pelvic pain was non-significantly more frequent in patients in groups 1 and 3 (Table IV).

Table IVDistribution of patients by group according to the presence or absence of pelvic pain

Pelvic pain	G1		G2		G3		p
	N	%	N	%	N	%	0,117
No	42	27,8%	12	19,7%	35	20,3%	
Yes	109	72,2%	49	80,3%	137	79,7%	

G1: ectopic pregnancy; G2: progressive intrauterine pregnancy; G3: non-progressive intrauterine pregnancy or failed pregnancy of undetermined location (GLI)

2.1.3. Metrorrhagia

Metrorrhagia was reported by 271 patients (70.6%). Metrorrhagia was significantly more frequent in patients in groups 1 and 3 (Table V).

Table VDistribution of patients by group according to the presence or absence of metrorrhagia

Bleeding	G1		G2		G3		P
	N	%	N	%	N	%	
No	44	29,1%	35	57,4%	34	19,8%	**0,048**
Yes	107	70,9%	26	42,6%	138	80,2%	

G1: ectopic pregnancy; G2: progressive intrauterine pregnancy; G3: non-progressive intrauterine pregnancy or failed pregnancy of undetermined location (GLI)

2.2. General physical examination

2.2.1. Hemodynamic constants

On admission, all patients were hemodynamically stable.

The distribution of blood pressure and heart rate values was similar in the different groups studied (Table VI).

Table VIDistribution of blood pressure and heart rate values by group

		Average	Standard deviation	Minimum	Maximum	P
TAS	G1	11,23	1,023	9	14	0,795
	G2	11,28	0,951	9	14	
	G3	11,18	1,057	9	15	
	Total	11,22	1,025	9	15	
TAD	G1	6,95	0,823	5	9	0,909
	G2	6,98	0,846	6	9	
	G3	6,93	0,823	5	9	
	Total	6,95	0,825	5	9	
FC	G1	79	8,2	60	109	0.397
	G2	79,9	8,1	68	108	
	G3	80,2	7,9	60	104	
	Total	79,6	8,0	60	109	

G1: ectopic pregnancy; G2: progressive intrauterine pregnancy; G3: non-progressive intrauterine pregnancy or failed pregnancy of undetermined location (GLI), SBP: systolic blood pressure, DBP: diastolic blood pressure, HR: heart rate.

2.2.3. Abdominal examination

Abdominal examination was normal in 327 patients (85.15%). Hypogastric tenderness was noted in 46 patients (12%). For the remaining 11 patients, the abdominal examination was not mentioned.

Abdominal examination data were comparable between the 3 groups studied (Table VII).

2.3 Gynaecological examination

2.3.1. Speculum examination

Speculum examination revealed endocavitary bleeding in 273 patients (71.3%) (Table VII).

2.3.2. The vaginal touch

On vaginal examination, uterine size was normal in most patients (99.2%), with the exception of 3 cases where the uterus appeared large, related to a myomatous uterus in all three patients.

We found no clinically palpable latero-uterine mass or pain in the vaginal pouches in any patient.

Comparing gynecological examination data between the 3 groups, we found no significant difference (Table VII).

Table VIIAbdominal and gynaecological examination data:

			Workforce	Percentage (%)	P
Abdominal examination	Without anomalies	G1	129	85,4	0,861
		G2	50	82	
		G3	148	86	
	Hypogastric sensitivity	G1	18	11 ,9	0,667
		G2	10	16,4	
		G3	18	10,5	
Gynaecological examination	Bleeding	G1	111	75	0,157
		G2	26	42,6	
		G3	136	81 ,4	
	Closed collar	G1	148	98	0,608
		G2	59	98,3	
		G3	143	99,3	
	Normal uterus	G1	148	98,7	0 ,954
		G2	57	98,3	
		G3	168	100	
	Enlarged uterus	G1	2	1,3	0 ,172
		G2	1	1,6	

| | G3 | 0 | 0 |

G1: ectopic pregnancy; G2: progressive intrauterine pregnancy; G3: non-progressive intrauterine pregnancy or failed pregnancy of undetermined location (GLI)

3. Further tests

3.1 Biological tests

3.1.1. Dodging of plasma ß-HCG

The median ß-HCG assay on admission was 666, ranging from 31.2 to 18,644 IU/ml.

After 48 hours, median ß-HCG was 655.45 ranging from 12 to 10125IU/ml (Table VIII).

Table VIIIDistribution of initial and 48-hour ß-HCG values

	Median	Minimum	Maximum
ß-HCG initial	666	31,2	18644
ß-HCG (48h)	655.45	12	10125

ß-HCG: Human chorionic gonadotropin

Initial ß-HCG levels were significantly higher in group 3 (p=0.001). The dosage after 48 h was higher in group 2, with no significant difference from the other groups (Table IX).

Table IXDistribution of initial and 48-hour mean ß-HCG values by group

	G1		G2		G3		P
	Median	[Q25, Q75]	Median	[Q25, Q75]	Median	[Q25, Q75]	
Initial ß-HCG	517	221-1097	602	369-958	1029	399-2640	**0,001**
ß-HCG at H 48	559	256-1200	1214	742-2042	499	182-1284	0,556

3.1.2. Blood count and haemostasis test

The blood count is not a diagnostic test, but is used to assess the patient's condition and detect anemia. The mean hemoglobin level was 12.05g/dl, with extremes ranging from 6.4g/dl to 15.6g/dl.

We noted that 149 cases (38.8%) had anemia on admission.

No patient presented with a haemostasis disorder on admission.

3.1.3. Number of ß-HCG assays before reaching final diagnosis

The average number of ß-HCG assays required to reach the final diagnosis was 2.39, with extremes ranging from 2 to 7 (Table X).

The mean number of ß-HCG assays was significantly higher in group 1, the EP group (p=0.012).

Table XDistribution of the number of ß -HCG assays by group

	Average	Standard deviation	Minimum	Maximum	P
G1	2,5	0,8	2	7	0,012
G2	2,39	0,6	2	4	
G3	2,28	0,6	2	5	
Total	2,39	0,7	2	7	

3.2. Pelvic ultrasound

3.2.1. Endometrial thickness

For endometrial thickness, there was a significant difference between the three groups.

Measurement of endometrial thickness was significantly higher in the G2 group (p<0.001) (Table XI).

Table XIDistribution of endometrial thickness on initial pelvic ultrasound by group

Endometrial thickness (mm)	Average	Standard deviation	Minimum	Maximum	P
G1	9,20	5,29	2	28	<0,001
G2	16,46	4,75	4	28	
G3	11,98	5,77	2	32	
Total	11,60	5,96	2	32	

G1: Ectopic pregnancy; G2: Progressive intrauterine pregnancy; G3: Non-progressive

intrauterine pregnancy or failed pregnancy of undetermined location (GLI); mm: Millimetre

3.2.2. Other ultrasound signs

Of the patients included, 37 had presented with a small effusion in the Cul de sac of Douglas. This finding was most frequently reported in the G1 group (p=0.006) (Figure 8).

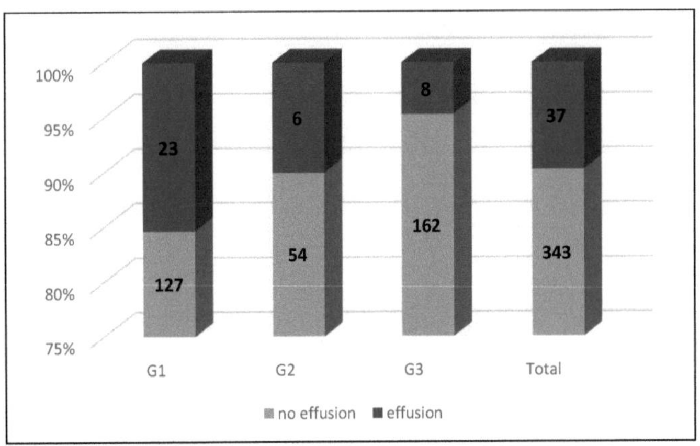

Figure 8Group distribution of intra-peritoneal effusion in the cul-de-sac of Douglas on initial pelvic ultrasound.

A corpus luteum was detected on ultrasound in 21 patients (5.5%). The presence of corpora lutea was more frequently reported in patients in the G1 group, although the difference was not statistically significant (p=0.554).

An ovarian cyst was detected in nine patients, with diameters ranging from 4 to 8 cm.

A myometrial image suggestive of uterine leiomyoma was found in 3 patients.

The average number of pelvic ultrasounds performed before reaching the final diagnosis was 1.93, with extremes ranging from 1 to 5. The number of ultrasounds required was significantly greater in group 2 (p<0.001) (table XII).

Table XIIDistribution of average number of ultrasound scans before reaching final diagnosis, by group

Average	Standard deviation	Minimum	Maximum	P

	Average	Standard deviation	Minimum	Maximum	P
G1	2,12	0,6	1	5	<0,001
G2	2,33	0,7	2	5	
G3	1,63	0,6	1	4	
Total	1,93	0,7	1	5	

G1: ectopic pregnancy; G2: progressive intrauterine pregnancy; G3: non-progressive

intrauterine pregnancy or failed pregnancy of undetermined location (GLI)

4. Management of pregnancies of undetermined location

4.1. Length of stay

The average hospital stay for our patients was 5.96 days, with extremes ranging from 3 to 20 days. It was significantly longer in group 1 (p<0.001).

Only one patient was hospitalized for 20 days. During her hospitalization, she underwent three ß -HCG determinations. The final outcome of her GLI was EP, initially treated with two doses of methotrexate, followed by radical laparoscopic surgical treatment for methotrexate failure.

Table XIII details the average length of hospital stay by group.

Table XIIIDistribution of average length of hospital stay for patients by group

	Average	Standard deviation	Minimum	Maximum	P
G1	9,53	3,9	4	20	<0,001
G2	3,9	1,2	3	7	
G3	3,67	1,1	3	8	
Total	5,96	3,8	3	20	

G1: ectopic pregnancy; G2: progressive intrauterine pregnancy; G3: non-progressive

intrauterine pregnancy or failed pregnancy of undetermined location (GLI)

4.2 Type of care

Uterine revision was performed as part of the diagnostic procedure in 10 patients (2.6%). The diagnosis was non-progressive GIU in 8 patients and EP in two.

Of the 151 patients in group G1 who were diagnosed with EP, medical management with methotrexate (MTX) was recommended in 125 cases (82.78%). Fifteen patients received two doses, and a single dose was administered to the remaining 110 patients.

Surgery was necessary in 40 patients (10.4%), either immediately in 26 or after failure of methotrexate in 14 (8 patients with unfavorable kinetics, two patients with a latero-uterine mass greater than 4cm, two fissure syndromes, one embryonic EP and one hemoperitoneum). The laparoscopic approach was adopted in all patients. Surgery was conservative in 3 cases (7%) and radical in 37 patients (93%).

The indications for surgery are detailed in the table below (Table XIV):

Table XIV Summary table of indications for surgical treatment of an EP

Indication for surgery	Workforce	Percentage (%)
Medium/large hemoperitoneum	4	10
MLU > 4 cm	6	15
Fissure syndrome	4	10
A failure of MTX	14	35
ß-HCG >5000 IU/L	1	2,5
Embryonic EP	2	5
Combining two indications Or more	9	22,5
Total	40	26,5

MLU: Lateral uterine mass; MTX: Methotrexate; ß-HCG: Human chorionic gonadotropin; EP: Extrauterine pregnancy; cm: centimeter.

Failed IUGs and GLI failures benefited from an expectant attitude with weekly monitoring of HCG levels until negativation. No patient progressed to gestational trophoblastic disease.

5. Performance of the HCG-ratio in predicting the outcome of pregnancies of undetermined location

An HCG-ratio between 0.87 and 1.66 had a concordance rate of 63.5% with the diagnosis of ectopic pregnancy (p<0.001), with a sensitivity (Se) of 79.3%, a specificity (Sp) of 84.5%, a positive predictive value (PPV) of 76.8% and a negative predictive value (NPV) of 86.4% (Table XV).

A ratio greater than 1.66 was significantly predictive of progressive pregnancy, with a kappa concordance rate of 0.791, a specificity of 91.5% and a PPV of 80.6%.

A ratio of less than 0.87 had a kappa concordance rate = 0.731 in the prediction of terminated pregnancy, a Se of 84.6% and a VPN of 99.1%.

Table XVPerformance of the HCG-ratio in predicting the final outcome of pregnancies of undetermined location

HCG- ratio / Final diagnosis	Threshold	Visit	Sp	VPP	VPN
Non-progressive intrauterine pregnancy Or Pregnancy with localization indeterminate stranded	<0.87	84.6	60.8	70.1	99.1
Ectopic pregnancy	0,87-1,66	79.3	84.5	76.8	86.4
Progressive intrauterine pregnancy	>1,66	26.4	91.4	80.6	47.9

Se: Sensitivity; Sp: Specificity; PPV: Positive predictive value; NPV: Negative predictive value

On the basis of our data, we have tried to establish new cut-offs for the HCG ratio combining the best compromise between sensitivity and NPV, in order to optimize its power to rule out the diagnosis of EP (Table XVI).

A ratio between 0.77 and 1.63 had a Se of 96% with a VPN of 95.6%.

Table XVI Performance of the new HCG-ratio thresholds in predicting the final outcome of pregnancies of undetermined location

HCG- ratio Final diagnosis	Threshold	Visit	Sp	VPP	VPN
Non-progressive intrauterine pregnancy **Or Pregnancy with localization indeterminate stranded**	≤0,77	80,23	92,89	90,2	85,2
Ectopic pregnancy	0,77-1.63	**96**	55,79	58,3	**95,6**
Progressive intrauterine pregnancy	>1,63	91,8	94,41	75,7	98,4

Se: Sensitivity; Sp: Specificity; PPV: Positive predictive value; NPV: Negative predictive value

6. Performance of the M4 model in predicting the outcome of pregnancies of undetermined location

Considering the 5% threshold for classifying women at high risk of EP, the M4 model had a Se of 59%, a Sp of 41.7%, a PPV of 40.2% and an NPV of 88.7% (Table XVII).

From our data, we tried to establish the threshold of the M4 model that associates the best compromise between Se and VPN. This threshold was 11%, with Se at 81%, Sp at 77%, PPV at 65% and NPV at 90% (Table XVII).

Table XVIIPerformance of the two thresholds of the M4 model in predicting the final outcome of pregnancies of undetermined location

Model M4 Threshold	Visit	Sp	VPP	VPN
5%	59	41.7	40.2	88.7
11%	81	77	65	90

Se: Sensitivity; Sp: Specificity; PPV: Positive predictive value; NPV: Negative predictive value

7. New predictive score for the outcome of pregnancies of undetermined location

In the light of our results, we established a new predictive score for EP in patients presenting with GLI, including as parameters the three variables significantly linked to EP risk in multivariate analysis, with their respective adjusted Odds ratios (Table XVIII).

Table XVIIIPrediction score for diagnosis of ectopic pregnancy

	P	OR	Coefficient	Confidence interval	
				Lower	Superior
HCG ratio between 0.78 and 1.63	<0,001	3,848	0-4	2,506	5,907
Initial ß-HCG >1000	0,017	1,975	0-2	1,130	3,453
Endometrial thickness < 10 mm	<0,001	1,279	0-1	1,211	1,352
Total score			**0 - 7**		

OR: Odds Ratio; ß-HCG: human chorionic gonadotropin; mm: millimeter

After applying this score to all the patients in our series, we retained the following results:

In our population, the mean was 3.3, with a standard deviation of 2.08 and extremes ranging from 0 to 7.

In group 1 (ectopic pregnancy), the mean score was 4.35, with a standard deviation of 1.86 and extremes ranging from 0 to 7.

In group 2 (progressive GIU), the mean was 2.48 with a standard deviation of 1.46 and extremes ranging from 0 to 7.

In group 3 (non-progressive intrauterine pregnancy or failed pregnancy of undetermined location), the mean was 2.74, with a standard deviation of 2.1 and extremes ranging from 0 to 7.

This score was significantly correlated with the risk of EP occurrence (p<0.001), with an area under the ROC curve (AUC) of 0.766 for a threshold of 3.5 (Figure 9). Patients with a score greater than or equal to 3.5 had a higher probability of EP with a sensitivity of 91%, specificity of 93%, PPV of 95% and NPV of 94%.

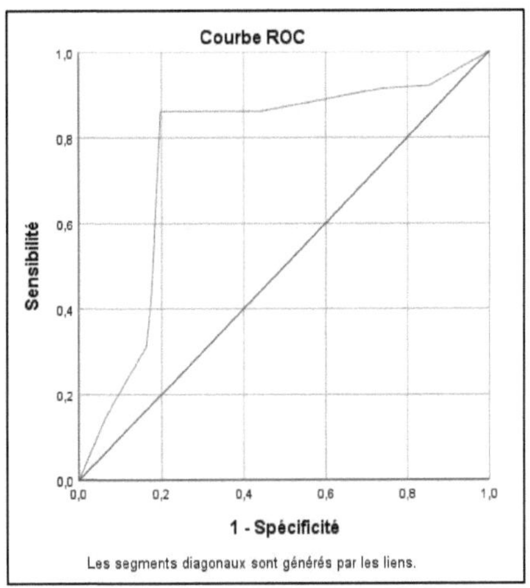

Figure 9ROC curve for the threshold value of 3.5 for the score predictive of ectopic pregnancy

8. Economic impact of applying the HCG-ratio and the M4 model

The actual cost of the diagnostic process leading to the final diagnosis was 356.38±141.45 dinars (DTN) per patient, with extremes ranging from 155-1002.5 DTN.

If the diagnostic approach followed the decision algorithm based on the HCG ratio (Figure 1), the average theoretical cost would have been 245.40±182.64 DTN [98.5-791.5] per patient, and we could have saved an average of 110.97 dinars per patient (Table XIX).

If the diagnostic approach followed the decision algorithm based on the M4 model (Figure 2), the average theoretical cost would have been 248.93±183.76 DTN [98.5-791.5] per patient, and we could have saved an average of 107.45 dinars per patient (Table XX).

Painting XIXDistribution of actual and estimated costs using the HCG ratio and the M4 model

	Mean ± standard deviation extremes	Savings
Actual cost	356,38±141,45 155-1002,5	-
Cost HCG ratio	245,40±182,64 98,5-791,5	110.97
Cost model M4	248,93±183,76 98,5-791,5	107.45

Comparing the estimated expenditure in the 3 groups, whatever the means of risk stratification adopted (HCG ratio or M4 model), the expected savings in group 2 (progressive intrauterine pregnancy) were significantly greater than in the other two groups.

Table XXBreakdown of HCG ratio and M4 model savings by group

Savings achieved		Average	Standard deviation	Minimum	Maximum	p
HCG ratio	G1	66,65	175,64	0	904	<0,001
	G2	207,56	101,01	0	489	
	G3	115,63	87,16	0	460	
	Total	110,97	139,08	0	904	
Model M4	G1	75,35	177,38	0	904	<0,001
	G2	180,82	110,10	0	489	

G3	109,60	84,19	0	345
Total	107,44	136,57	0	904

G1: ectopic pregnancy; G2: progressive intrauterine pregnancy; G3: non-progressive intrauterine pregnancy or failed pregnancy of undetermined location (GLI)

If we were to calculate the expected savings after excluding group 1 patients (EP), the HCG ratio predictions would save an average of 221 dinars (98.5-904 dinars) per patient, and those of the M4 Model would save an average of 202.25 dinars (98.5-904 dinars) per patient.

DISCUSSION

1. Epidemiological data

1.1 Incidence and prevalence of pregnancy of undetermined location

Several studies have attempted to estimate the incidence and prevalence of pregnancy of undetermined location.

In fact, the prevalence of GLI is variable because it depends on several parameters, including the variability of diagnostic criteria and definitions, and above all the quality of the ultrasound examination, which in turn depends on the skill of the sonographer and the performance of the equipment used. [9].

The prevalence of GLI is estimated by most authors at 8-10% of young pregnancies with pathological onset [[3,4]

According to data from a prospective study conducted in the United Kingdom over a 12-month period and including 6201 first-trimester pregnant women, the GLI rate was 10.9%. [4].

In one of the first published works on GLI, Banerjee et al reported a rate of GLI at 8% of pregnancies presumed pathological at their onset [110] .

In our series, the annual incidence of GLI was estimated at an average of 55 cases/year, representing a prevalence of 1.4%. This rate is low compared with the literature, and can be explained by late consultations, often leading to a diagnosis of certainty as to the location of the pregnancy as early as the first consultation.

1.2. Maternal age

Maternal age does not appear to be an important factor in the GLI study. According to the authors, it varies between 31 and 32.8 years of age [111, 6, ,112].

In our study, the age group most frequently affected was 31 to 35 years old, with an average age of 32.8±5.7 years and extremes ranging from 18 to 46 years, which coincides with the data in the literature (Table XXI). This could be explained by the fact that this age group is that of women at the height of their genital activity.

Table XXISummary table of maternal age in the literature

Author	Banerjee [111]	Bobdiwala [[6]	Fistouris [1[12]	Our study
Year of study	2001	2020	2022	2023
Type of study	Foresight	Multicenter prospective study	Retrospective cohort	Retrospective
Number of patients	104	3272	1061	384
Average age (years)	31	32	31	32,8
Age limits (years)	17-45		15-49	18-46

Maternal age has been considered by some authors for the prediction of GLI evolution. It was most often higher in the GLI group than in the other groups [1[11, 113].

A comparative study of the three groups according to age showed that in our series, the age of patients in the G1 and G3 groups was significantly higher than in the G2 group (p=0.042), which is in line with the literature.

1.3 Gender and parity

According to the results of Banerjee et al, the mean gestational age in women consulting for GLI was 3.2 with extremes ranging from 1 to 9, with no significant difference between the different groups (p= 0.879). [111].

Florio et al, in a prospective study carried out in 2007 and including 536 patients diagnosed with GLI, found that the majority of patients had a gestité greater than or equal to 3. The parity of the different categories according to GLI outcome was also comparable [1[13].

In our series, gestational age was 3±1.8, with no significant difference (p=0.317) between groups. Our results are therefore consistent with those reported in the literature.

Few authors have studied parity as a predictor of GLI outcome. According to the data of Florio et al, the patients included were mostly pauci pares, without parity having any predictive value for the outcome of GLI [113].

In our study, the mean parity of our patients was 1.38±1.1, with extremes ranging from 0 to 5. The parity of women with progressive intrauterine pregnancy was significantly lower than the other groups (p=0.008).

2. Risk factors for EP in the case of GLI

2.1. History of ectopic pregnancy

A history of EP is considered an important risk factor for EP recurrence. [114,15].

This fact has been underlined by the results of several authors.

Karaer et al, in a prospective case-control study investigating risk factors for the occurrence of ectopic pregnancy in Turkey, concluded that a previous EP was the most important etiological factor, with an adjusted odds ratio (AOR) of recurrence of 13.1 [16].

On the other hand, Ashraf Moini et al have shown that a history of EP significantly increases the risk of subsequent EP (OR = 17.16, CI [1.89-155.67], *P* = 0.01).[17].

In a prospective cohort carried out between January 2010 and June 2017 and including 217 women who had had an ectopic pregnancy, 41 women or 18.9% had a recurrence of EP within the following five years [18].

In our study, a history of EP was found in 11.3% of cases in patients who had progressed to EP (group G1), with a significant difference from the other groups (p=0.032), reinforcing the data in the literature.

2.2. Previous caesarean section

The link between a history of caesarean delivery and the risk of EP remains debated.

In a retrospective cohort of 260,249 women, Bowman et al concluded that a history of two or three caesarean sections is considered a risk factor for subsequent ectopic pregnancy. [19]. The results published by E Hemminki et al also support this finding [2[20].

However, Cheng LI points out in his results that a history of caesarean section has no effect on the risk of EP. [221].

In our study, comparing the 3 groups according to cesarean section history, we found no significant difference (p=0 .597).

2.3. Previous abdomino-pelvic surgery

The role of abdomino-pelvic surgery as a risk factor for EP is much debated in the literature [2[22].

In our series, 27 patients (6.6%) had a history of pelvic surgery other than caesarean section, including 10 in group G1.

No significant relationship was found between previous pelvic surgery and the risk of EP (p=0.443).

Our results were consistent with those of Rachdi et al, who found that 7% of patients treated for EP in the obstetrics and gynaecology department of Monastir had undergone pelvic surgery. [223].

In a review of the literature published in 2014, Elraiyah et al focused on a history of appendectomy as a risk factor for EP [224].

While other authors, such as Mannistö et al ,in a cohort study including 23,997 women who had undergone appendectomy, concluded that the latter did not increase the risk of EP [25].

In our series, we found no statistically significant relationship between history of appendectomy and risk of EP (p=0.406).

2.4. Previous tubal plasty

Tubal surgery is recognized as a risk factor for EP [22]. This may be explained by the reduction in tubal motility and the peritoneotubal adhesions it engenders [26].

In a review of the literature published in 2015, Taran et al found that a history of tubal surgery significantly increased the risk of EP with an Odd ratio greater than 4 [27].

Our results were in perfect agreement with the literature, given that tubal plasty was significantly correlated with a risk of EP (p=0.008).

2.5. History of infertility

Several authors have concluded that the risk of EP increases in women with a history of infertility [[16,21,28].

In a case-control study involving 803 cases of EP and 1683 controls (pregnancies carried to term), Bouyer et al showed that ovulation stimulation with clomiphene citrate was associated with a risk of ectopic pregnancy in univariate analysis, but this association disappeared after adjustment for prior infertility. A history of infertility was strongly associated with the risk of ectopic pregnancy, with a dose-response relationship and an adjusted odds ratio for infertility of more than 2 years of 2.7 (95 percent CI: 1.8, 4.2) [29].

However, the frequency of infertility in the population of women with EP varies widely in the literature, from 3.1 to 30%.

In our study, only 4.2% of women had a history of infertility, with a significant difference in favor of those in the EP group (0.028) (Table XXII).

Table XXII Frequency of infertility in cases of ectopic pregnancy in the literature

Authors	Country	Year	Frequency
Li.C [21]	Shanghai	2015	16.74 %
Garbin.O [[30]	France	2010	17.32 %
Basnet.R [3[31]	Nepal	2015	13 %
Ferkous.G [3[32]	Morocco	2011	5.1 %
Moini.A [[17]	Iran	2014	30 %
Ayadi.J [33]	Tunisia (Sfax)	2006	9.9 %
Dimassi [[34]	Tunisia (Mahdia)	2016	3.1 %
Our study	Tunisia (Ben Arous)	2024	4.2 %

2.6. History of upper genital infection

Upper genital infection (UGI), through the tubal lesions it causes, is one of the most important risk factors for EP. [222 ,35] .

Chlamydia trachomatis being the most frequently incriminated germ [[36].

Following the introduction of screening and treatment campaigns for Chlamydia infection in Uppsala County, Sweden, Egger et al observed a significant drop in the rate of ectopic pregnancies. [37].

A study carried out by Mol al in the Netherlands between 1980 and 2005 showed that the peak in the incidence of chlamydia trachomatis infections in 1983 was followed by a peak in the incidence of EP in 1988. [338].

In our series, a history of IGH was found in only 6 patients. Indeed, this low number may be the reason why IGH does not appear to emerge as a significant risk factor for the occurrence of EP (p=0.552).

2. 7. Contraception

The use of contraceptives reduces the total incidence of unplanned pregnancies, whether intrauterine or extrauterine. [39].

Schultheis et al, in **a** prospective cohort study including 9,256 patients with different contraceptive methods observed over a period of 2 to 3 years ,estimated that the incidence of EPU is lower in the groups of women using contraception compared with women using no contraception or barrier contraception. [440].

Whereas in the case of contraceptive failure, this risk is greater in women **using** intrauterine devices (IUDs), microprogestins or tubal sterilization as a means of **contraception** [41].

In our series, IUD and microprogestin use do not appear to be associated with the risk of EP in women presenting initially for GLI.

2.8. Smoking

Maternal smoking is a risk factor widely studied in epidemiology and potentially associated with the occurrence of an ectopic pregnancy. [442].

This could be explained by the harmful and toxic effects of nicotine on tubal function [222].

In a case-control study conducted in Washington, Stergachis et al studied the incidence of smoking in 274 patients who had presented with an EP, comparing them with 727 patients of childbearing age. Smoking women were found to have a higher risk of EP than non-smoking women (OR=1.3). [443].

Saraiya et al found equivalent results. In fact, the risk of having an EP was increased by 1.9 in women who smoked [444].

Of the 384 cases studied in our series, 43 patients were smokers, representing 11.19% of cases. However, smoking was not associated with the risk of EP in our study population (p=0.679), probably due to the low proportion of women who smoked.

3. Clinical study

3.1. Amenorrhea

In a study conducted in Sweden over a three-year period and including 915 women with GLI, the authors found that the average duration of amenorrhea varied between 39 and 46 days. This duration was higher in the non-progressive intrauterine pregnancy group [7].

In a prospective study of 1625 patients published by Banerjee et al, the mean duration of amenorrhea ranged from 32.5 to 52 days [111].

Our results were close to those reported in the literature. Indeed, the mean duration of amenorrhea was 6.37 weeks (44.59 days) and was significantly longer in the non-progressive intrauterine pregnancy and GLI failure group (p<0.001).

3.2. Breakthrough bleeding

According to Condous et al, only 26% of women with GLI did not present with vaginal bleeding. For patients who presented to the gynaecological emergency department with metrorrhagia, the final outcome of their GLI was often a failed UGI [9].

According to the results of our study, metrorrhagia was reported by 271 patients (70.6%). They were significantly more frequent in patients with EP or arrested/failed UGI (groups 1 and 3) (p=0.048).

3.3. Pelvic pain

Condous et al, in a prospective study conducted in 2005 concluded that among 527 cases of GLI analyzed, 59% were asymptomatic while 48% presented with pelvic pain [9].

In our study, 295 patients (76.82%) presented with pelvic pain on admission. They were more frequent in patients in groups 1 and 3, but not significantly so (p=0.117).

4. Further tests

4.1 Pelvic ultrasound

Today, the improved performance of ultrasound scanners used in gynecology departments has had a major impact on medical practice in obstetrics and gynecology.

In fact, the combination of suprapubic and endovaginal ultrasound, the diagnostic performance of ultrasound and the expertise of the sonographer are important elements that improve the sensitivity of ultrasound and the early detection of ultrasound signs leading to a diagnosis of certainty. [9 ,45] .

In the series by Emma Kirk et al, published in 2007 on 5318 cases attending a specialist early gestation unit in London, endovaginal ultrasound revealed GLI in 4693 cases (89.6%) and EP in 91 (1.7%). Only 456 women (8.7%) were classified as GLI [46].

On the other hand, this study reported that endovaginal ultrasonography has a sensitivity of 73.9% (95% CI: 65.1-81.6) , with a specificity of 99.9% (95% CI: 99.8-100), a PPV of 96.7% (95% CI: 90.7-99.3) and a NPV of 99.4% (95% CI: 99.2-99.6) in the diagnosis of an EP [46].

The search for an intrauterine gestational sac or a latero-uterine mass constitutes two crucial steps in the practice of suprapubic and endovaginal ultrasonography in the case of GLI. [47].

In the course of a normal intrauterine pregnancy, the following structures begin to be visualized in the uterine cavity in succession: a gestational sac at four and a half weeks' amenorrhea, the umbilical vesicle, the first embryonic structure, at around five weeks' amenorrhea, an embryo at five and a half weeks' amenorrhea, followed rapidly by cardiac activity [48].

Several studies have investigated the correlation between endometrial thickness and the evolution of GLI.

Spandofer et al. concluded that, in patients whose final GLI outcome was an EP, the endometrium was thinner on initial ultrasound compared with other patients who had a different outcome [449].

Moschos et al found that an initially thickened endometrium is strongly associated with UGI [550].

Our results were in perfect agreement with the literature: endometrial thickness was significantly higher in the progressive GIU group (G2) (p<0.001).

4.2. Plasma ß- HCG assay

To this day, HCG continues to be the most widely used biochemical marker in routine practice for monitoring GLI [551].

In a GLI population, a single serum HCG assay is not sufficient to predict the final outcome of a GLI. However, it is of interest in determining the threshold value of plasma HCG above which an intrauterine gestational sac should be visualized on suprapubic and/or endovaginal ultrasound (EEV). This so-called "discriminative HCG" value is used to identify patients at high risk of EP and depends essentially on the resolution of the EEV, the experience of the sonographer and the HCG kit used by the laboratory. [[8, 552] .

Currently, thanks to the improved resolution of EEV, the discriminatory level of serum HCG required to identify an intrauterine pregnancy on ultrasound is set at between 1500 and 2500 IU/l [553].

However, this threshold sometimes gives a false sense of security to the practitioner, who tends to underestimate the concern of localizing a pregnancy when levels are well below the adopted values, and consequently misses the risks incurred in the event of extra-uterine localization. On the other hand, a pregnancy may not be identified despite its intra-uterine location and a serum ß-HCG level exceeding the predefined threshold.

This fact was underlined by Kirk et al, who showed, by comparing the hormonal behaviour of EPs diagnosed on initial endovaginal ultrasound with those initially classified as GLI, that the median plasma HCG level retained for the latter was 635 IU/l, i.e. below the discriminatory threshold. [[54].

In our study, the mean initial plasma HCG level was 901 IU/l in patients whose final GLI outcome was an EP.

Conversely, some progressive UGI are not visualized on initial ultrasound even with plasma HCG levels above discriminatory values [551].

In a retrospective study published in 2014, the authors concluded that in some cases ultrasound identification of a GIU is only possible from very high plasma HCG levels [55].

Other studies, such as Doubilet [56] and Connolly [57] agree with the precipitous results.

Multiple pregnancies, endometrial polyps, uterine fibroids, adenomyosis and obesity are just some of the factors involved. [5[51, 55].

Thus, a non-interventional attitude with ß-HCG kinetics seems defensible in hemodynamically stable patients in order to avoid a possible misdiagnosis.

Kader et al were the first to study the hormonal profile in early pregnancy. They concluded that during progressive GIU, plasma HCG levels increase by 66% or more over 48 hours. [58]. In 2004, Barnhart et al suggested an increase of at least 53% over 48 hours [59].

More recently, in a cohort of 1249 patients, the authors proposed with a CI of 99.9 a minimum increase of 35% in the case of progressive GIU [660].

It should be noted that this increase in plasma HCG levels during progressive GIU also varies according to the initial level of this hormone. Thus, when initial HCG is above 3000 mIU/mL, it increases by 33%,40% for initial HCG values between 1500 and 3000 mIU/mL and 49% for initial concentrations below 1500 mIU/mL [551].

On the other hand, some authors have also studied plasma HCG kinetics during spontaneously resolved GLI.

Barnhart et al found that plasma HCG levels decline by 21 to 35% at 48 hours in cases of spontaneously resolved GLI or failed GLI. They also concluded that this decline is more rapid for higher initial HCG values [661].

Unfortunately, this hormonal behavior does not appear to be unambiguous in predicting the diagnosis of an EP in a GLI population. According to Silva et al, the hormonal profile of an EP can mimic progressive GLI or complete spontaneous abortion in 29% of cases [662].

In our work, the initial ß-HCG level was significantly higher in the arrested/failed GIU group (p=0.001). Dosing after 48 h was higher in the progressive GIU group, with no significant difference from the other groups.

4.3. Plasma progesterone level

The corpus luteum, placenta and adrenal glands are the source of serum progesterone, a natural progestogen whose role is crucial for maintaining pregnancy. [551].

The association of progesterone and plasma ß-HCG levels strongly predicts the final outcome of GLI. Plasma progesterone levels <20 nmol/L are strongly associated with spontaneous resolution of GLI, while levels >25 nmol/L help predict viable GLI. For serum progesterone levels >60nmol/l , the most likely diagnosis is progressive UGI. That said, progesterone levels provide information on the viability of the pregnancy without refining the investigation of localization [663].

In this context, Bobdiwala et al have shown that the probability of a viable pregnancy is strongly associated with high serum progesterone levels [2].

Indeed, the probability of progressive UGI increased from 0.0001 to 0.097 for serum progesterone values ranging from 0 to 20 nmol/L [2].

A meta-analysis including 26 studies published in 1998 concluded that a single plasma progesterone value was sufficient to predict the non-viability of a pregnancy, regardless of the site. [[64].

Our study did not take into account the serum progesterone level on admission, as this biological parameter is difficult to access in an emergency in our context.

5. GLI coverage

5.1. Surgical treatment of GLI

Some authors, such as Barnhart et al, agree that uterine curettage in order to differentiate between an EP and an arrested GIU seems legitimate in certain contentious cases before resorting to medical treatment with methotrexate [[65].

According to Pisarska et al, uterine curettage may be recommended provided that the possibility of progressive UGI has been ruled out either by serum progesterone determination (≤15-9 nmol/L) or by the non-ascendance of plasma ß-HCG levels at 48 hours [66].

Thus, a decrease of at least 15% in plasma ß-HCG levels in the 24 hours following uterine curettage would favour the diagnosis of a non-advanced GIU, whereas stagnation or an increase in the latter would argue in favour of EP as the most likely diagnosis, and the patient would be managed as an EP carrier. [551].

However, for Condous et al, uterine curettage does not appear to be indicated in the diagnostic approach to GLI [667].

In our study, 10 uterine curettages were performed for diagnostic purposes (2.6%). The diagnosis was non-progressive UGI in 8 patients and EP in two.

5.2. Medical treatment of GLI with methotrexates

Methotrexate (MTX) has been used in cases of persistent GLI in clinically stable patients with suspected EP. Depending on patient preference, MTX may be offered as an alternative to uterine evacuation. This is a folic acid antagonist that has a high success rate in selected cases of EUS [68]. A dose of 50 mg/m^2 of MTX is administered intramuscularly, and if HCG does not decrease by at least 15% between days 4ème and 7ème , then the same dose of MTX can be repeated [69]. As with uterine revision, before administering MTX, care must be taken to ensure that the pregnancy is not a progressive intrauterine pregnancy. Unfortunately, misdiagnosis has been described, leading to congenital malformations, abortions and elective termination of pregnancy. [770,771].

A prospective multicenter study randomly selected 73 hemodynamically stable patients diagnosed with EP with HCG levels below 1,500 mIU/mL or diagnosed with GLI with HCG levels below 2,000 mIU/mL or who had plateau HCG levels. A total of 41 patients received MTX (1 mg/kg intramuscularly), and 32 women were monitored without MTX administration. In this study, MTX was not superior to expectant treatment in cases of EP or GLI with low or plateau HCG titers [772].

Recently, cases classified as GLI and initially treated with MTX but who actually had HCG-producing tumors (i.e. gestational and non-gestational choriocarcinomas) have been described [773,74]. Although rare, this possibility must be taken into account, as incorrect diagnosis can delay appropriate treatment and create resistance to the chemotherapeutic agent.

Unfortunately, there is no consensus regarding follow-up and timing of intervention in GLI. Our protocol is based on an HCG discriminant value of 3,500 mIU/mL and a variation in HCG titres at 48 hours.

5.3. Therapeutic abstention

Given that spontaneous regression of EPs is possible and is seen in approximately 20% of cases [2[22]abstention from treatment can be proposed for patients with easy access to emergency care. These women should be asymptomatic, with a plasma HCG level below 1000 mIU/ml and an initial pelvic ultrasound without abnormalities [75].

In our series, failed UGIs and GLI failures benefited from an expectant attitude with weekly monitoring of HCG levels until negativation. No patient progressed to gestational trophoblastic disease.

6. Predicting the final outcome of GLI

Pregnancy with indeterminate location is a term that was first introduced by the Royal College of Obstetricians and Gynaecologists in October 2006 to describe the clinical situation in which a pregnancy test is positive while no signs in favour of EP or IUP are identified on EVT [76].

While awaiting a final diagnosis, these patients undergo a range of clinical, biological and ultrasound examinations. Thus, the evolution of GLI can be favorable towards an intrauterine pregnancy (IUP) or a failed GLI, or unfavorable towards a persistent GLI or an ectopic pregnancy (EP) (Figure 10).[[1].

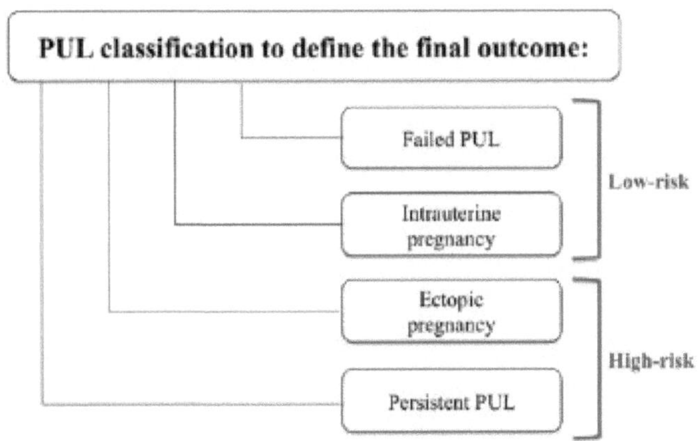

Figure 10Classification of pregnancies with undetermined location according to final diagnosis. [[1]

Today's endovaginal ultrasound probes are increasingly efficient, enabling us to visualize very young pregnancies in the vast majority of cases. Nevertheless, there are still cases of early pregnancy where neither an EP nor a miscarriage can be confirmed: these are pregnancies of undetermined location, which are on the increase. [6,77,78,79].

This is often due to women seeking care as soon as pregnancy tests are positive, especially if they have undergone medically assisted reproduction. [54].

The extra-uterine localization of a pregnancy remains the obsession of every practitioner. Indeed, the importance of this quest stems from the often underestimated frequency of EPs, on the one hand, and the severe repercussions of neglecting this pathology, on the other. [114].

According to a meta-analysis published in 2012, 7 to 20% of women with pregnancies of undetermined location will have an EP as their final outcome [78].

In fact, in a multicenter study including 1962 patients who consulted a gynecological emergency room for GLI, the diagnosis of EP was reported in 8 to 16% of cases. [80].

In our study, of the 384 women included, 151 (39.3%) had a final diagnosis of EP. This rate was relatively higher than those found in the literature. This may be explained by the frequency of risk factors for EP in our study population.

Thus, the authors set out to develop ways of sorting patients according to the degree of suspicion of a high-risk EP. This enabled them to better manage healthcare expenditure without compromising the quality of care for patients with a high suspicion of ectopic pregnancy. [5]. The most commonly used parameters are serum progesterone, the HCG ratio, the M4 model and, more recently, the M6 model, which includes serum progesterone. The HCG ratio is the most commonly adopted method. A number of mathematical models were then developed with a view to improving the management of GLI.

In our work, we have decided to study the HCG ratio and the M4 Model, as they are the most suitable for our conditions of exercise.

6.1. Performance of the HCG Ratio in predicting the outcome of pregnancies of undetermined location

The HCG Ratio is calculated by dividing the plasma ß- HCG assay by the assay performed 48 hours previously. Various thresholds have been established to predict the final outcome of GLI. According to British guidelines, an HCG above 1.63 indicates a progressive GLI, whereas a ratio below 0.5 classifies the GLI as a non-progressive pregnancy. For patients with a ratio between 0.5 and 1.63, they are classified at high risk of ectopic pregnancy and require more careful monitoring [81]. As for American recommendations, a non-progressive pregnancy is suspected by an HCG ratio of less than 1.33 to 1.53, depending on the value of initial plasma ß-HCG [8[82,883]French guidelines classify a GLI as a presumed non-progressive pregnancy if the HCG ratio is below 0.85, provided that the initial plasma ß-HCG value is below 2000 IU/L. [884].

This level of heterogeneity between guidelines is of concern when they can be used to determine the viability of a desired pregnancy or to rule out the diagnosis of an EP. Hence, we proposed to study the performance of the HCG ratio using the thresholds adopted in the most recent data in the literature, and to determine our own thresholds. In our work, we considered that an HCG ratio value below 0.87 corresponds to a failed GLI, a value above 1.66 to a possible UGI and a ratio between 0.87 and 1.66 to a probable EP. [3,85].

These same thresholds were used by Izhar et al in their prospective study published in 2022. The authors found that the HCG ratio had a sensitivity (Se) of 72%, a specificity (Sp) of 73%, a positive predictive value (PPV) of 44% and a good negative predictive value (NPV) of 90% for EP. [5]. These results are comparable to those published by Nadim et al in 2019 [886].

In a prospective multicenter study published in 2021, Bobdiwala et al found that the higher the HCG ratio, the greater the probability of an evolutive pregnancy. Thus, for an HCG ratio threshold of less than 0.8, the probability of a progressive UGI is less than or equal to 0.001, whereas it is 0.883 for a ß-HCG ratio of 4. [2].

Bignardi et al concluded in their prospective observational study that the HCG ratio is higher in the case of an evolutive GIU than in the case of a non evolutive pregnancy with a Sn 77.2%, a Sp 95.8%, a VPP 86.6%, a VPN 90.9%. They also reported that an HCG ratio greater than 2 increased the probability that the intrauterine pregnancy was progressive. [87].

According to the results of Condous et al, for an HCG ratio of less than 0.87, the Se and Sp for the detection of a non-progressive GIU were 93.1% and 90.8 %, respectively [88].

A meta-analysis published in 2018 and including 8 studies evaluating the performance of the HCG ratio in GLI triage, concluded that it performed better than simple ß-HCG assays in predicting the viability of a GLI but not as well in predicting its location [79].

In our study, a ratio below 0.87 had a kappa concordance rate = 0.731 in the prediction of terminated pregnancy, with a Se of 84.6% and a VPN of 99.1%. An HCG-ratio between 0.87 and 1.66 had a concordance rate of 63.5% with the diagnosis of ectopic pregnancy (p<0.001) with a Se of 79.3%, a Sp of 84.5%, a PPV of 76.8% and a negative predictive value NPV of 86.4%. We were also able to establish new thresholds with a better compromise between sensitivity and specificity for the diagnosis of EP: a ratio between 0.77 and 1.63 had a Se of 96% with a VPN of 95.6. Our results thus concur with those of the literature.

6.2. Performance of the M4 model in predicting the outcome of pregnancies of undetermined location

Although some teams continue to use the HCG ratio to triage patients presenting with GL, the multiplication of proposed thresholds makes some practitioners wary of adopting it in their day-to-day practice. In this context, several mathematical models have been developed to optimize the management of GLI, such as the M4 model. [77].

For risk stratification of pregnancies of undetermined location, the M4 model takes into account two parameters: the initial plasma HCG value and the HCG ratio. Thus, in a given GLI population, women will be classified as "high risk" if the probability of having an EP is ≥5%, and as "low risk" of EP for a probability <5%. [77].

Several authors have studied the performance of the M4 model in predicting the risk of EP. Van Claster et al have shown that using the M4 mathematical model to triage patients with GLI reduces follow-up by 70%, with a good NPV of around 97.5%. [80].

According to the results of Izhar et al, in a GLI population, the M4 model predicts the risk of EP with a Se of 86 .4%, a Sp of 91% ,a VPN of 95.8 % and VPP of 76 % [5].

In a multicenter study including 1271 cases of GLI, Guha et al concluded that 84% of EPs were initially classified as high-risk pregnancies by the M4 with an OR of 19.4 (11.5-32.8) [89][.

Bobdiwala et al showed in a multicenter prospective cohort conducted in 2016 that the M4 mathematical model correctly classified low-risk GLI in 97% of cases and high-risk GLI in 82%. Moreover ,they concluded that using the M4 the area under the curve to differentiate an EP from an evolutive or non evolutive GLI is 0.84 [77].

In an Australian study published in 2020, the authors showed that in predicting high-risk pregnancies the M4 model has a Se of 80.0% (95% CI 71.1 to 86.5%), a Sp of 75.9% (95% CI 72.2 to 79.3%), a PPV of 37.8% (95% CI 33.8 to 42.1%) and an NPV 95.3% (95% CI 93.1 to 96.9%) [90].

In our work, considering the 5% threshold for classifying women at high risk of EP, the M4 model had a Se of 59%, an Sp of 41.7%, a PPV of 40.2% and an NPV of 88.7%. These values were well below the performance of the M4 model found in the literature. This could be explained by the ethnic and socio-demographic differences of the populations studied. We were therefore able to improve the Model's performance in our population by setting the cut-off at 11%, which gave a Se of 81%, a Sp of 77%, a PPV of 65% and a NPV of 90% (Table XXIII).

Table XXIII Performance of the M4 model in predicting the outcome of pregnancies of undetermined location in the literature

Author	Year	Type of study	Sensitivity	Specific	VPP	VPN
Van Claster et al [80]	2013	Retrospective multicenter	88%	69,9%	20,4%	97,5%
Bobdiwala et al [77]	2016	Multicenter prospective study	82%	70%	23%	97%

Nadim et al [90]	2020	Single-center retrospective	80%	75,9%	37,8%	95,3%
Izhar et al [5]	2022	Single-center retrospective	86,4%	91%	76%	95,8%
Our series	2024	Single-center retrospective	59%	41,7%	40,2%	88,7%

PPV: Positive Predictive Value/NPV: Negative Predictive Value

6.3. HCG ratio versus M4 model in predicting the outcome of pregnancies of undetermined location

The HCG ratio and the M4 Model have made it possible to optimize GLI monitoring and have revolutionized care for the women concerned.

Several authors have therefore compared the performance of the HCG ratio and the M4 model, in order to adopt the most suitable method for predicting the final outcome of GLI in a given population.

For Bobdiwala et al, the M4 model is superior to the HCG ratio in terms of predicting GLIs at high risk of EP. [77].

A recent meta-analysis published in 2018 concluded that the M4 model was the best tool for predicting an EP by comparing it to the HCG ratio and serum progesterone measurement alone [79].

Guha et al in their multicenter study involving 1271 cases of GLI, also concluded that M4 is superior to HCG ratio and serum progesterone measurement alone in predicting ectopic pregnancy [889].

However, most authors agree that the HCG ratio was better at predicting the viability of a GLI and worse at assessing the risk of EP. Indeed, according to a meta-analysis published by Bobdiwala et al, for the prediction of the final outcome of GLI in progressive UGI, the area under the curve for the HCG ratio was 0.97 (95% CI 0.87-0.99) while that for the M4 Model was 0.86. Similarly for persistent or progressive GLI, with an area under the curve of 0.98 for the HCG ratio versus 0.84 for the M4 model [79].

At the end of this comparison, it appears that the M4 model is better at predicting the final outcome of a GLI in EP. However, the HCG ratio is the best means of predicting the viability or otherwise of a GLI.

6.4. Performance of the M6 Model in predicting the outcome of pregnancies of undetermined location

A new mathematical model has been developed to predict the final outcome of GLI: the M6 Model. [5, 551]. This model takes into account the HCG ratio as well as initial progesterone and ß-HCG levels [8].

As with the M4 model, the M6 model could be integrated into diagnostic strategies for GLI, including two-step decision algorithms or the "two-step approach" proposed by Van Calster et al. [991] (Figure 11).

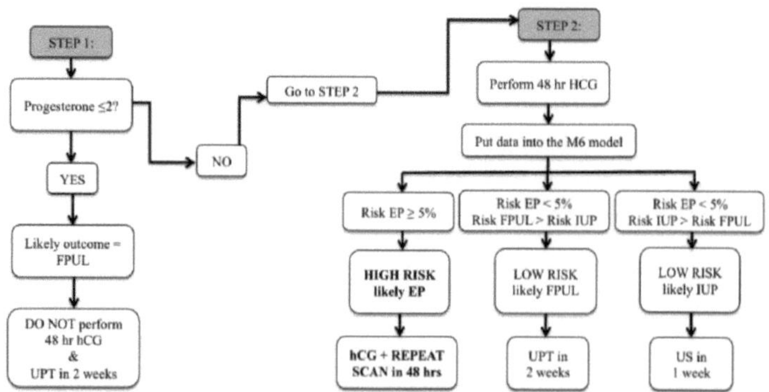

Figure 11Two-stage decision algorithm proposed by Van Calster et al. [991].

The M6 Model has undergone several external validations and its performance in predicting the outcome of GLI has been demonstrated by several authors [1,92,93].

According to a French study published in 2022, EPs were correctly classified by the M6 model with a sensitivity of 96.4% and a negative predictive value of 98.9%. [8].

In our study, the M6 model was not evaluated, as serum progesterone levels are not usually measured in emergency situations under our conditions of practice.

7. New markers in the management of GLI

Several studies have evaluated serum levels of numerous biomarkers such as cancer antigen 125 (CA125) , creatine kinase (CK) and inhibin A in predicting the final outcome of GLI [551].

Indeed, Condous et al concluded in a prospective study published in 2005 that serum CA125 and CK levels do not predict the outcome of GLI. As for the CA125 ratio (CA125 at 48h /CA125 at 0h), if incorporated into a logistic regression model, it can give an indication of the evolutivity of GLI. Its ineffectiveness in detecting GLI at high risk of EP limits its clinical usefulness. [9[94].

In the same vein, Chetty et al have shown the relative usefulness of serum inhibin A assay in differentiating spontaneously resolved GLI from progressive GLI. Indeed, a serum inhibin A level ≤ 11 pmol/L is in favor of a failed GLI. However, progesterone continues to be the only and best biomarker for predicting GLI evolutivity [995].

Based on our results, we were able to propose a new predictive score for the outcome of GLI integrating the parameters usually used in the initial assessment of our patients: HCG ratio, initial ß-HCG level and endometrial thickness. This score showed very promising results, with a sensitivity of 91%, specificity of 93%, PPV of 95% and NPV of 94% for a score above 3.5.

8. Economic impact of applying the HCG-ratio and the M4 model

All the proposed models for predicting the outcome of GLI are presumed to be beneficial in terms of triaging women presenting to gynaecological emergency departments. The lower the suspicion of EP, the less investigations are required. In a country where healthcare is expensive, such a strategy would be fruitful. In addition, follow-ups can be strategic, allowing women deemed to be at high risk to benefit from all the necessary care [5].

However, given the variability of discriminative thresholds, external validation of these models in different ethnic groups is necessary in order to homogenize the management of GLI by following universal decision-making algorithms [551].

In our study, considerable savings could have been made according to the predictions of the HCG ratio and the M4 Model, particularly in low-risk groups: 221 dinars (98.5-904 dinars) per patient for the HCG ratio and 202.25 dinars (98.5-904 dinars) per patient for the M4 Model.

9. Strengths and limitations of our work

Pregnancy of undetermined location (GLI) represents a diagnostic and management challenge for the practitioner, faced with asymptomatic patients at risk of life-threatening ectopic pregnancy (EP). The use of mathematical models to stratify the risk of ectopic pregnancy at the first consultation may avoid hospitalization of patients considered to be "low risk", thus saving these women a particularly anxiety-provoking situation and generating savings in terms of healthcare costs. With this in mind, we decided to carry out this retrospective descriptive and analytical study to assess the performance of the M4 model and the HCG ratio in risk stratification of pregnancies of undetermined location (GLI).

The strengths of our study were:

- Our study is of crucial medical importance in Tunisia. Indeed, no national study has evaluated the use of these means in the triage of GLI under our skies.
- As women become increasingly educated, the rapid diagnosis of pregnancy often leads to very early and untimely consultations, making this an ever topical issue.
- We feel that the population studied in our work is considered a fairly representative sample, which has had a real impact on the statistical power of the study.
- We have used the most recent valuation methods that are best suited to our operating conditions: the HCG ratio and the M4 Model.
- According to our literature review, this is the first study to evaluate the economic impact of using mathematical models in the triage of patients with GLI.

However, it is important to recognize the inherent limitations of this work:

- Monocentricity
- Collecting and analyzing files retrospectively can lead to errors and biases in the analysis of statistical results.

- The new M6 mathematical model used to predict the final outcome of GLI has not been evaluated, as serum progesterone levels are not readily available in our emergency setting.
- We have not addressed the question of the psychological impact on these women awaiting localization of pregnancy which, beyond the devastating effect, could lead to anxiety disorders during the course of an eventual intrauterine pregnancy.

10. Outlook and recommendations

10.1. Recommendations

In light of the results of our study, we can propose the following algorithms for stratifying the evolutive risk of GLI (Figures 12,13,14).

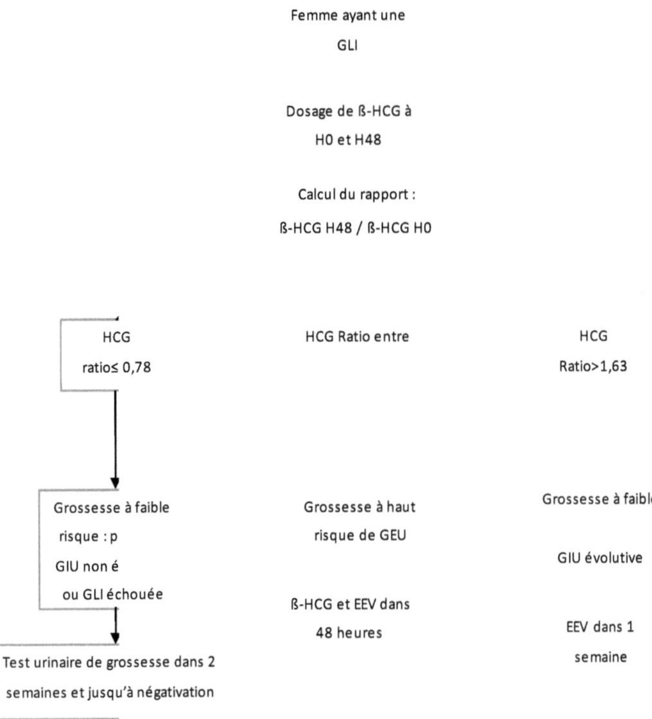

Figure 12GLI management algorithm based on risk stratification using the new HCG ratio thresholds

GIU: Intrauterine pregnancy; GLI: Pregnancy of undetermined location; EEV: Endovaginal ultrasound; GEU: Extrauterine pregnancy; ß -HCG: Human chorionic gonadotropin.

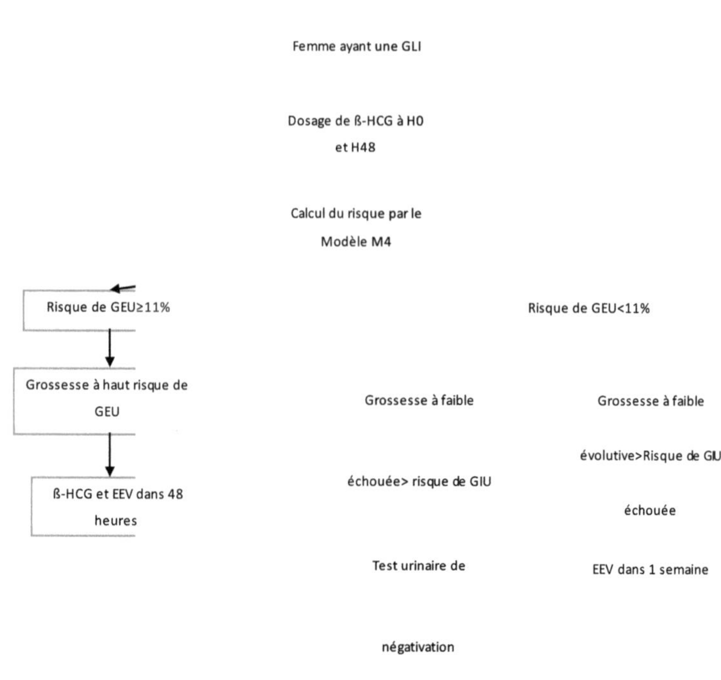

Figure 13GLI management algorithm based on risk stratification using the new M4 thresholds

GIU: Intrauterine pregnancy; GLI: Pregnancy of undetermined location; EEV: Endovaginal ultrasound; GEU: Extrauterine pregnancy; ß -HCG: Human chorionic gonadotropin.

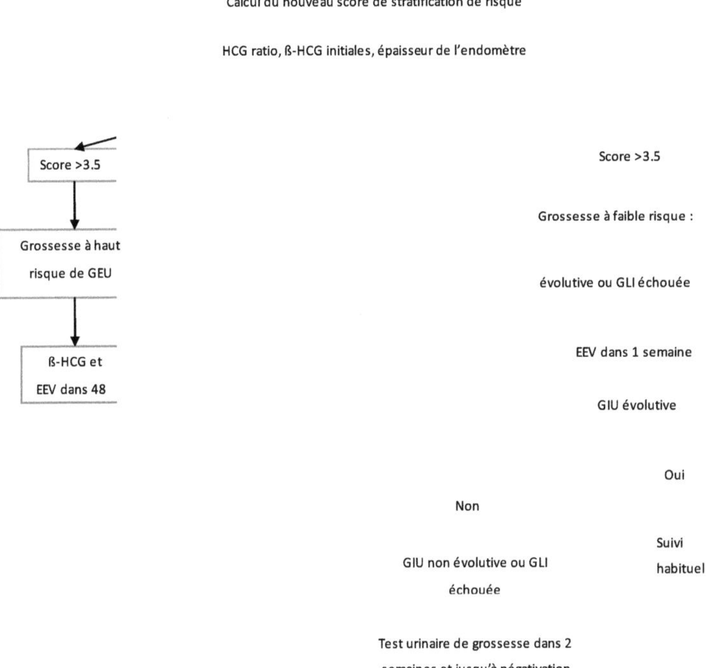

Figure 14GLI management algorithm based on the new risk stratification score

GIU: Intrauterine pregnancy; GLI: Pregnancy of undetermined location; EEV: Endovaginal ultrasound; GEU: Extrauterine pregnancy; ß -HCG: Human chorionic gonadotropin.

10.2. Outlook

A prospective multicenter study may be proposed to assess the performance of the new HCG ratio cut-offs and the M4 model in GLI risk stratification.

In this way, management algorithms more suited to our population can be developed, with more attentive follow-up for women at high risk of EP.

Furthermore, taking into account statistically significant parameters, we propose to use our new score integrating the HCG ratio with thresholds of 0.78 and 1.63, initial ß-HCG assay and endometrial thickness measurement in prospective multicenter studies in order to validate it and adjust its positivity threshold.

CONCLUSIONS

Pregnancy of undetermined location (GLI) refers to the situation in which a woman has a positive urine or blood pregnancy test, but cannot locate her pregnancy on pelvic ultrasound.

The aim of our study was to evaluate the performance of the M4 model and the HCG ratio in risk stratification of pregnancies with indeterminate location (GLI) through a retrospective study of a series of 384 patients with GLI (January 2017 to April 30, 2023).

The mean age of our patients was 32.8±5.7 years, with extremes ranging from 18 to 46 years, and 34.4% of patients were over 35 years of age (n=132).

The mean gestational age of our patients was 3±1.8 and mean parity 1.38±1.1.

The main risk factors for EP presented by our patients were: Previous EP (11.3%), previous tubal plasty (4%) and previous infertility (6%).

No significant differences were observed when comparing gynecological examination data between the 3 groups.

The median ß-HCG assay was 666 IU/ml on admission and 655.45 IU/ml after 48 hours. The initial ß-HCG level was significantly higher in group 3 (p=0.001) and the dosage after 48 h was higher in group 2, with no significant difference from the other groups.

The average number of ß -HCG assays before reaching the final diagnosis was 2.39, with the G1 group requiring the highest number of assays (p=0.012).

For pelvic ultrasound, endometrial thickness was highest in the G3 group and lowest in the G1 group (p<0.001).

The average number of scans required before final diagnosis was 1.93 scans. Group G2 required the highest number of scans (p<0.001).

As for GLI management, the average length of hospital stay for patients was 5.96 days, with extremes ranging from 3 to 20 days. It was higher in the G1 group (p<0.001).

EP was diagnosed in 151 patients. Medical management with methotrexate was reported in 125 cases (82.78%). Fifteen patients received two doses, and a single dose was sufficient for the remaining 110 patients. Surgery was required in 40 patients (10.4%).

For the HCG ratio, the best Se (84.6%) and VPN (99.1%) were seen in the group of non-progressive intrauterine pregnancies or failed indeterminate-location pregnancies (HCG ratio <0.87). Progressive intrauterine pregnancies (HCG ratio >1.66) had the highest Sp (91.4%) and PPV (80.6%). For the diagnosis of EP (HCG ratio between 0.87 and 1.66), the performance parameters of the HCG ratio were as follows: Se (79.3%), Sp (84.5%), PPV (76.8%) and NPV (86.4%).

Based on our data, we were able to establish new cut-offs for the HCG ratio combining the best compromise between sensitivity and NPV, in order to optimize its power to rule out the diagnosis of EP. Thus, a ratio between 0.77 and 1.63 had a Se of 96% with a VPN of 95.6% in predicting the risk of EP.

Considering the 5% threshold for classifying women at high risk of EP, the M4 model had a Se of 59%, a Sp of 41.7%, a PPV of 40.2% and an NPV of 88.7%.

From our data, we were able to establish the threshold of the M4 model that associates the best compromise between Se and VPN. This threshold was 11%, with Se at 81%, Sp at 77%, PPV at 65% and NPV at 90%.

In the light of our results, we established a new score predictive of EP in patients presenting for GLI, including as parameters the three variables significantly linked to EP risk on multivariate analysis, assigning them respectively as coefficients their adjusted Odds ratios: an HCG ratio between 0.78 and 1.63 (OR: 3.848), initial ß-HCG >1000 IU/L (OR: 1.975) and endometrial thickness < 10 mm (OR: 1.279). This score showed promising performance in predicting the risk of GLI: sensitivity 91%, specificity 93%, PPV 95% and NPV 94%.

In terms of healthcare costs, we have shown that the use of the HCG ratio and the M4 Model would result in significant savings without affecting patient prognosis.

Certainly, the prevalence of GLI is constantly increasing, given the over-medicalization of pregnancy and conception, particularly in the context of medically assisted reproduction. The final outcome of a GLI as an EP is not negligible, with the possibility of rupture. Outpatient diagnostic management would be feasible after risk stratification using the HCG ratio and the M4 Model, adapting their thresholds to our context, and why not develop new scores adapted to our population and practice conditions.

REFERENCES

1. **Bobdiwala S, Al-Memar M, Farren J, Bourne T.** Factors to consider in pregnancy of unknown location. *Womens Health (Lond)* *2017;13:2733-.*

2. **Bobdiwala S, Kyriacou C, Christodoulou E, Farren J, Mitchell-Jones N, Al-Memar M, et al.** Evaluating cut-off levels for progesterone, β human chorionic gonadotropin and β human chorionic gonadotropin ratio to exclude pregnancy viability in women with a pregnancy of unknown location: A prospective multicenter cohort study. *Acta Obstet Gynecol Scand 2021;101:4655-.*

3. **Kirk E, Condous G, Van Calster B, Van Huffel S, Timmerman D, Bourne T.** Rationalizing the follow-up of pregnancies of unknown location. *Hum Reprod 2007;22:174450-.*

4. **Cordina M, Schramm-Gajraj K, Ross JA, Lautman K, Jurkovic D.** Introduction of a single visit protocol in the management of selected patients with pregnancy of unknown location: a prospective study. *BJOG 2011;118: 6937-.*

5. **Izhar R, Husain S, Tahir MA, Ala SH, Imtiaz R, Husain S, et al.** Triaging women with pregnancy of unknown location: evaluation of protocols based on single serum progesterone, serum hCG ratios, and model M4. *J Reprod Infertil 2022;23:10713-.*

6. **Bobdiwala S, Christodoulou E, Farren J, Mitchell-Jones N, Kyriacou C, Al-Memar M, et al.** Triaging women with pregnancy of unknown location using two-step protocol including M6 model: clinical implementation study. *Ultrasound in Obstet Gynecol* 2020;55:10514-.

7. **Fistouris J, Bergh C, Strandell A.** Classification of pregnancies of unknown location according to four different hCG-based protocols. *Hum Reprod 2016;31: 220311-.*

8. **Dap M, Chaillot M, Rouche J, Mezan de Malartic C, Morel O.** Retrospective evaluation of a decision support algorithm for pregnancies of undetermined location. *Gynecol Obstet Fertil Senol 2022;50:390-4.*

9. **Condous G, Kirk E, Lu C, Van Huffel S, Gevaert O, De Moor B, et al.** Diagnostic accuracy of varying discriminatory zones for the prediction of ectopic pregnancy in women with a pregnancy of unknown location. *Ultrasound Obstet Gynecol 2005;26:7705-.*

10. **Banerjee S, Aslam N, Zosmer N, Woelfer B, Jurkovic D.** The expectant management of women with early pregnancy of unknown location. *Ultrasound Obstet Gynecol 1999;14:2316-.*

11. **Banerjee S, Aslam N, Woelfer B, Lawrence A, Elson J, Jurkovic D.** Expectant management of early pregnancies of unknown location: a prospective evaluation of methods to predict spontaneous resolution of pregnancy. *BJOG 2001;108:15863-.*

12. **Fistouris J, Bergh C, Strandell A.** Pregnancy of unknown location: external validation of the hCG-based M6NP and M4 prediction models in an emergency gynaecology unit. *BMJ Open 2022;12:e058454.*

13. **Florio P, Severi FM, Bocchi C, Luisi S, Mazzini M, Danero S, et al.** Single serum activin a testing to predict ectopic pregnancy. *J Clin Endocrinol Metab 2007;92:174853-.*

14. **Hendriks E, Rosenberg R, Prine L.** Ectopic pregnancy: diagnosis and management. *Am Fam Physician 2020;101:599-606.*

15. **Farquhar CM.** Ectopic pregnancy. *Lancet 2005;366:58391-.*

16. **Karaer A, Avsar FA, Batioglu S.** Risk factors for ectopic pregnancy: a case-control study. *Aust N Z J Obstet Gynaecol 2006;46:521-7.*

17. **Moini A, Hosseini R, Jahangiri N, Shiva M, Akhoond MR.** Risk factors for ectopic pregnancy: A case-control study. *J Res Med Sci 2014;19:8449-.*

18. **Ellaithy M, Asiri M, Rateb A, Altraigey A, Abdallah K.** Prediction of recurrent ectopic pregnancy: A five-year follow-up cohort study. *Eur J Obstetrics Gynecol Reprod Biol 2018;225:708-.*

19. **Bowman ZS, Smith KR, Silver RM.** Cesarean delivery and risk for subsequent ectopic pregnancy. *Am J Perinatol 2015;32:815.*

20. **Hemminki E, Meriläinen J.** Long-term effects of cesarean sections: ectopic pregnancies and placental problems. *Am J Obstet Gynecol 1996;174:156974-.*

21. **Li C, Zhao WH, Zhu Q, Cao SJ, Ping H, Xi X, et al.** Risk factors for ectopic pregnancy: a multi-center case-control study. *BMC Pregnancy Childbirth 2015;15:187.*

22. **Gervaise A, Fernandez H.** Diagnostic and therapeutic management of ectopic pregnancies. *J Gynecol Obstet Biol Reprod (Paris) 2010;39: F1724-.*

23. **Rachdi R, Fekih MA, Hajjami R, Messaoudi L, Chibani M, Brahim H.** La grossesse extra-uterine à propos de 70 observations. *Med Maghreb 1991;28:9-12.*

24. **Elraiyah T, Hashim Y, Elamin M, Erwin PJ, Zarroug AE.** The effect of appendectomy in future tubal infertility and ectopic pregnancy: a systematic review and meta-analysis. *J Surg Res 2014;192:368-74.*

25. **Männistö J, Sammalkorpi H, Niinimäki M, Mentula M, Mentula P.** Association of complicated appendicitis on the risk of later in vitro fertilization treatment requirement and ectopic pregnancy: a nationwide cohort study. *Acta Obstet Gynecol Scand 2021;100:14906-.*

26. **Poncelet É, Leconte C, Fréart-Martinez É, Laurent N, Lernout M, Bigot J, et al.** Ultrasound and MRI appearance of ectopic pregnancy. *Imag Femme 2009;19:1718-.*

27. **Taran FA,Kagan KO, hubner M,Hoopmann M,Wallwiener D,Brucker S.**The Diagnosis and Treatment of Ectopic Pregnancy.Deutshes Arzteblatt International.oct2015.112(41) :693-703*

28. **Rana P, Kazmi I, Singh R, Afzal M, Al-Abbasi FA, Aseeri A, et al.** Ectopic pregnancy: a review. *Arch Gynecol Obstet 2013;288:74757-.*

29. **Bouyer J, Coste J, Shojaei T, Pouly JL, Fernandez H, Gerbaud L, et al.** Risk factors for ectopic pregnancy: a comprehensive analysis based on a large case-control, population-based study in France. *Am J Epidemiol 2003;157:18594-.*

30. **Garbin O, Helmlinger C, Meyer N, David-Montefiore E, Vayssiere C.** Can 74% of ectopic pregnancies be treated with medical therapy? About a series of 202 patients. *J Gynecol Obstet Biol Reprod (Paris) 2010; 39:-306.*

31. **Basnet R, Pradhan N, Bharati L, Bhattarai N, Basnet BB, Sharma B.** To determine the risk factors associated with ectopic pregnancy. *Asian J Pharm Clin Res 2015;8:937-.*

32. **Ferkous G.** Ectopic pregnancy: about 117 cases [Thesis]. *Rabat: Université Mohamed V, Faculté de Médecine et de Pharmacie; 2011*

33. **Ayadi J.** Grossesse extra-utérine: aspects épidémiologiques cliniques et thérapeutiques à propos de 112 cas [Thesis]. *Sfax: Université de Sfax, Faculté de Médecine; 2006.*

34. **Dimassi R.** Ectopic pregnancy: epidemiological, diagnostic and therapeutic aspects: about 128 cases. *Monastir: University of Monastir, Faculty of Medicine; 2016.*

35. **Derniaux E, Lucereau-Barbier M, Graesslin O.** Follow-up and counseling after upper genital infections. *J Gynecol Obstet Biol Reprod (Paris) 2012;41:9229-.*

36. **Shaw JLV, Wills GS, Lee KF, Horner PJ, McClure MO, Abrahams VM, et al.** Chlamydia trachomatis infection increases Fallopian tube PROKR2 via TLR2 and NFκB activation resulting in a microenvironment predisposed to ectopic pregnancy. *Am J Pathol 2011;178:25360-.*

37. **Egger M, Low N, Smith GD, Lindblom B, Herrmann B.** Screening for chlamydial infections and the risk of ectopic pregnancy in a county in Sweden: ecological analysis. *BMJ 1998;316:177680-.*

38. **Mol F, van Mello NM, Mol BW, van der Veen F, Ankum WM, Hajenius PJ.** Ectopic pregnancy and pelvic inflammatory disease: a renewed epidemic? *Eur J Obstet Gynecol Reprod Biol 2010;151:1637-.*

39. **Rosenthal MA, McQuillan SK.** Contraception in adolescent girls. *CMAJ 2021;193:E14756-.*

40. **Schultheis P, Montoya MN, Zhao Q, Archer J, Madden T, Peipert JF.** Contraception and ectopic pregnancy risk: a prospective observational analysis. *Am J Obstet Gynecol 2021;224:2289-.*

41. **Furlong LA.** Ectopic pregnancy risk when contraception fails. A review. *J Reprod Med 2002;47:8815-.*

42. **Dekeyser-Boccara J, Milliez J.** Tobacco and ectopic pregnancy: is there a causal link? *J Gynecol Obstet Biol Reprod (Paris) 2005;34:11923-.*

43. **Stergachis A, Scholes D, Daling JR, Weiss NS, Chu J.** Maternal cigarette smoking and the risk of tubal pregnancy. *Am J Epidemiol 1991;133:3327-.*

44. **Saraiya M, Berg CJ, Kendrick JS, Strauss LT, Atrash HK, Ahn YW.** Cigarette smoking as a risk factor for ectopic pregnancy. *Am J Obstet Gynecol 1998;178:4938-.*

45. **Mathlouthi N, Olfa S, Fatnassi A, Ben Temime R, Makhlouf T, Attia L, et al.** Ultrasound diagnosis of ectopic pregnancy: Prospective study about 200 cases. *Tunis Med 2013;91:2547-.*

46. **Kirk E, Papageorghiou AT, Condous G, Tan L, Bora S, Bourne T.** The diagnostic effectiveness of an initial transvaginal scan in detecting ectopic pregnancy. *Hum Reprod 2007;22:28248-.*

47. **Drobny J.** Sonography in the management of symptomatic pregnancies of unknown location. *Bratisl Lek Listy 2008;109:2549-.*

48. **Hôpital Necker Enfants Malades.** Ultrasound: from month to month. *[Online]. [Accessed 18/01/2024], available at URL: https://maternite-necker.aphp.fr/echographie-mois-en-mois/*

49. **Spandorfer SD, Barnhart KT.** Endometrial stripe thickness as a predictor of ectopic pregnancy. *Fertil Steril 1996;66:4747-.*

50. **Moschos E, Twickler DM.** Endometrial thickness predicts intrauterine pregnancy in patients with pregnancy of unknown location. *Ultrasound Obstet Gynecol 2008;32:929-34.*

51. **Pereira PP, Cabar FR, Gomez ÚT, Francisco RP.** Pregnancy of unknown location. *Clinics (Sao Paulo) 2019;74:e1111.*

52. **Menard JP, Bretelle F, D'Ercole C, Boubli L.** Place of biology among diagnostic strategies for ectopic pregnancy. *Immunoanal Biol Spec 2011;26:-138.*

53. **Seeber BE, Barnhart KT.** Suspected ectopic pregnancy. *Obstet Gynecol 2006;107(2 Pt 1):399413-.*

54. **Kirk E, Daemen A, Papageorghiou AT, Bottomley C, Condous G, De Moor B, et al.** Why are some ectopic pregnancies characterized as pregnancies of unknown location at the initial transvaginal ultrasound examination? *Acta Obstet Gynecol Scand 2008;87:11504-.*

55. **Ko JKY, Cheung VY.** Time to revisit the human chorionic gonadotropin discriminatory level in the management of pregnancy of unknown location. *J Ultrasound Med 2014;33:46571-.*

56. **Doubilet PM, Benson CB.** Further evidence against the reliability of the human chorionic gonadotropin discriminatory level. *J Ultrasound Med 2011;30: 163742-.*

57. **Connolly A, Ryan DH, Stuebe AM, Wolfe HM.** Reevaluation of discriminatory and threshold levels for serum β-hCG in early pregnancy. *Obstet Gynecol 2013;121:65.*

58. **Kadar N, Caldwell BV, Romero R.** A method of screening for ectopic pregnancy and its indications. *Obstet Gynecol 1981;58:162.*

59. **Barnhart KT, Sammel MD, Rinaudo PF, Zhou L, Hummel AC, Guo W.** Symptomatic patients with an early viable intrauterine pregnancy: hCG curves redefined. *Obstet Gynecol 2004;104:50.*

60. **Seeber BE, Sammel MD, Guo W, Zhou L, Hummel A, Barnhart KT.** Application of redefined human chorionic gonadotropin curves for the diagnosis of women at risk for ectopic pregnancy. *Fertil Steril 2006;86:4549-.*

61. **Barnhart K, Sammel MD, Chung K, Zhou L, Hummel AC, Guo W.** Decline of serum human chorionic gonadotropin and spontaneous complete abortion: defining the normal curve. *Obstet Gynecol 2004;104(5 Pt 1):97581-.*

62. **Silva C, Sammel MD, Zhou L, Gracia C, Hummel AC, Barnhart K.** Human chorionic gonadotropin profile for women with ectopic pregnancy. *Obstet Gynecol 2006;107:605.*

63. **Kirk E, Condous G, Bourne T.** Pregnancies of unknown location. *Best Pract Res Clin Obstet Gynaecol 2009;23:4939-.*

64. **Mol BW, Lijmer JG, Ankum WM, van der Veen F, Bossuyt PM.** The accuracy of single serum progesterone measurement in the diagnosis of ectopic pregnancy: a meta-analysis. *Hum Reprod 1998;13:3220-7.*

65. **Barnhart KT, Katz I, Hummel A, Gracia CR.** Presumed diagnosis of ectopic pregnancy. *Obstet Gynecol 2002;100:50510-.*

66. **Pisarska MD, Carson SA, Buster JE.** Ectopic pregnancy. *Lancet 1998;351: 111520-.*

67. **Condous G, Kirk E, Lu C, Van Calster B, Van Huffel S, Timmerman D, Bourne T.** There is no role for uterine curettage in the contemporary diagnostic workup of women with a pregnancy of unknown location. *Hum Reprod 2006;21:2706-10.*

68. **American College of Obstetricians and Gynecologists.** ACOG Practice Bulletin No. 94: Medical management of ectopic pregnancy. *Obstet Gynecol 2008;111:147985-.*

69. **Stovall TG, Ling FW, Gray LA.** Single-dose methotrexate for treatment of ectopic pregnancy. *Obstet Gynecol 1991;77:7547-.*

70. **Usta IM, Nassar AH, Yunis KA, Abu-Musa AA.** Methotrexate embryopathy after therapy for misdiagnosed ectopic pregnancy. *Int J Gynaecol Obstet 2007; 99:2535-.*

71. **Nurmohamed L, Moretti ME, Schechter T, Einarson A, Johnson D, Lavigne SV, et al.** Outcome following high-dose methotrexate in pregnancies misdiagnosed as ectopic. *Am J Obstet Gynecol 2011;205:533.e1-3.*

72. **van Mello NM, Mol F, Verhoeve HR, van Wely M, Adriaanse AH, Boss EA, et al.** Methotrexate or expectant management in women with an ectopic pregnancy or pregnancy of unknown location and low serum hCG concentrations? A randomized comparison. *Hum Reprod 2013;28:607-.*

73. **Larish A, Kumar A, Kerr S, Langstraat C.** Primary gastric choriocarcinoma presenting as a pregnancy of unknown location. *Obstet Gynecol 2017;129: 2814-.*

74. **McCarthy CM, Unterscheider J, Burke C, Coulter J.** Metastatic gestational choriocarcinoma: a masquerader in obstetrics. *Ir J Med Sci 2018;187:1279-.*

75. **Gervaise A.** Conduct in nonsurgical management of ectopic pregnancy. *Rev Sage Femme 2004;3:2131-.*

76. **Condous G, Timmerman D, Goldstein S, Valentin L, Jurkovic D, Bourne T.** Pregnancies of unknown location: consensus statement. *Ultrasound Obstet Gynecol 2006;28:121-2.*

77. **Bobdiwala S, Guha S, Van Calster B, Ayim F, Mitchell-Jones N, Al-Memar M, et al.** The clinical performance of the M4 decision support model to triage women with a pregnancy of unknown location as at low or high risk of complications. *Hum Reprod 2016;31:142535-.*

78. **van Mello NM, Mol F, Opmeer BC, Ankum WM, Barnhart K, Coomarasamy A, et al.** Diagnostic value of serum hCG on the outcome of pregnancy of unknown location: a systematic review and meta-analysis. *Hum Reprod Update 2012;18:60317-.*

79. **Bobdiwala S, Saso S, Verbakel JY, Al-Memar M, Van Calster B, Timmerman D, et al.** Diagnostic protocols for the management of pregnancy of unknown location: a systematic review and meta-analysis. *BJOG 2019;126: 1908-.*

80. **Van Calster B, Abdallah Y, Guha S, Kirk E, Van Hoorde K, Condous G, et al.** Rationalizing the management of pregnancies of unknown location: temporal and external validation of a risk prediction model on 1962 pregnancies. *Hum Reprod 2013;28:60916-.*

81. **National Institute for Health and Care Excellence (NICE).** Ectopic pregnancy and miscarriage: diagnosis and initial management. *London: NICE; 2023.*

82. **American College of Obstetricians and Gynecologists.** ACOG Practice Bulletin No. 193: Tubal Ectopic Pregnancy. *Obstet Gynecol 2018;131:e91103-.*

83. **Practice Committee of American Society for Reproductive Medicine.** Medical treatment of ectopic pregnancy: a committee opinion. *Fertil Steril 2013;100:638-44.*

84. **Huchon C, Deffieux X, Beucher G, Capmas P, Carcopino X, Costedoat-Chalumeau N, et al.** Pregnancy loss: French clinical practice guidelines. *Eur J Obstet Gynecol Reprod Biol 2016;201:1826-.*

85. **Condous G, Van Calster B, Kirk E, Timmerman D, Van Huffel S, Bourne T.** Prospective cross-validation of three methods of predicting failing pregnancies of unknown location. *Hum Reprod 2007;22:1156-60.*

86. **Nadim B, Leonardi M, Infante F, Lattouf I, Reid S, Condous G.** Rationalizing the management of pregnancies of unknown location: Diagnostic accuracy of human chorionic gonadotropin ratio-based decision tree compared with the risk prediction model M4. *Acta Obstet Gynecol Scand 2020;99:38190-.*

87. **Bignardi T, Condous G, Alhamdan D, Kirk E, Van Calster B, Van Huffel S, et al.** The hCG ratio can predict the ultimate viability of the intrauterine pregnancies of uncertain viability in the pregnancy of unknown location population. *Hum Reprod 2008;23:19647-.*

88. **Condous G, Kirk E, Van Calster B, Van Huffel S, Timmerman D, Bourne T.** General obstetrics: Failing pregnancies of unknown location: a prospective evaluation of the human chorionic gonadotrophin ratio. *BJOG 2006;113:5217-.*

89. **Guha S, Ayim F, Ludlow J, Sayasneh A, Condous G, Kirk E, et al.** Triaging pregnancies of unknown location: the performance of protocols based on single serum progesterone or repeated serum hCG levels. *Hum Reprod 2014;29: 93845-.*

90. **Nadim B, Leonardi M, Stamatopoulos N, Reid S, Condous G.** External validation of risk prediction model M4 in an Australian population: Rationalising the management of pregnancies of unknown location. *Aust N Z J Obstet Gynaecol 2020;60:92834-.*

91. **Van Calster B, Bobdiwala S, Guha S, Van Hoorde K, Al-Memar M, Harvey R, et al.** Managing pregnancy of unknown location based on initial serum progesterone and serial serum hCG levels: development and validation of a two-step triage protocol. *Ultrasound Obstet Gynecol 2016;48:6429-.*

92. **Bobdiwala S, Christodoulou E, Farren J, Mitchell-Jones N, Kyriacou C, Al-Memar M, et al.** Triaging women with pregnancy of unknown location using two-step protocol including M6 model: clinical implementation study. *Ultrasound Obstet Gynecol 2020;55:10514-.*

93. **Christodoulou E, Bobdiwala S, Kyriacou C, Farren J, Mitchell-Jones N, Ayim F, et al.** External validation of models to predict the outcome of pregnancies of unknown location: a multicentre cohort study. *BJOG 2021;128: 55262-.*

94. **Condous G, Kirk E, Syed A, Van Calster B, Van Huffel S, Timmerman D, et al.** Do levels of serum cancer antigen 125 and creatine kinase predict the outcome in pregnancies of unknown location? *Hum Reprod 2005;20:334854-.*

95. **Chetty M, Sawyer E, Dew T, Chapman AJ, Elson J.** The use of novel biochemical markers in predicting spontaneously resolving "pregnancies of unknown location". *Hum Reprod 2011;26:131823-.*

96. **Barnhart K, van Mello NM, Bourne T, Kirk E, Van Calster B, Bottomley C, et al.** Pregnancy of unknown location: a consensus statement of nomenclature, definitions, and outcome. *Fertil Steril 2011;95:85766-.*

APPENDICES

Appendix 1: Classification of the final outcome of pregnancies with indeterminate location. [96]

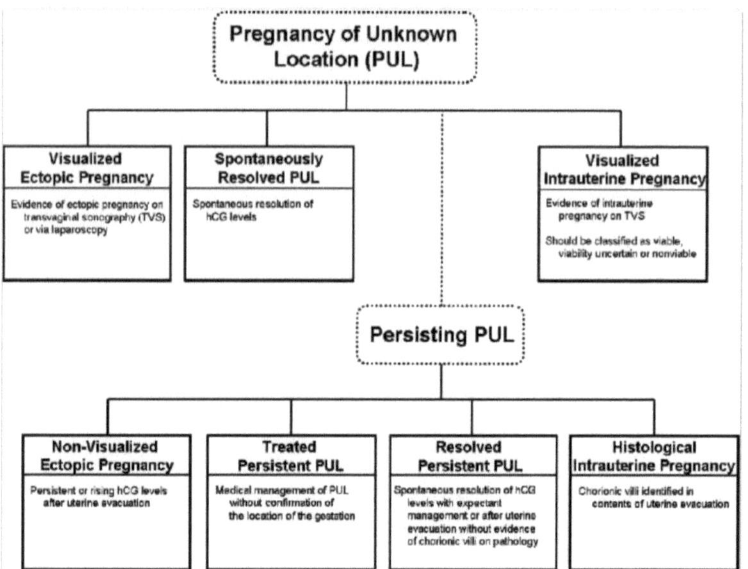

<table>
<tr><td>Likely
failed PUL</td><td>Likely
ectopic/ PPUL</td><td>Likely
ongoing IUP</td></tr>
<tr><td>hCG ratio
<0.87</td><td>hCG ratio
$\geq$0.87
and $\leq$1.66</td><td>hCG ratio
>1.66</td></tr>
</table>

Appendix 3: Risk stratification of indeterminate pregnancies using the M4 mathematical model [80]

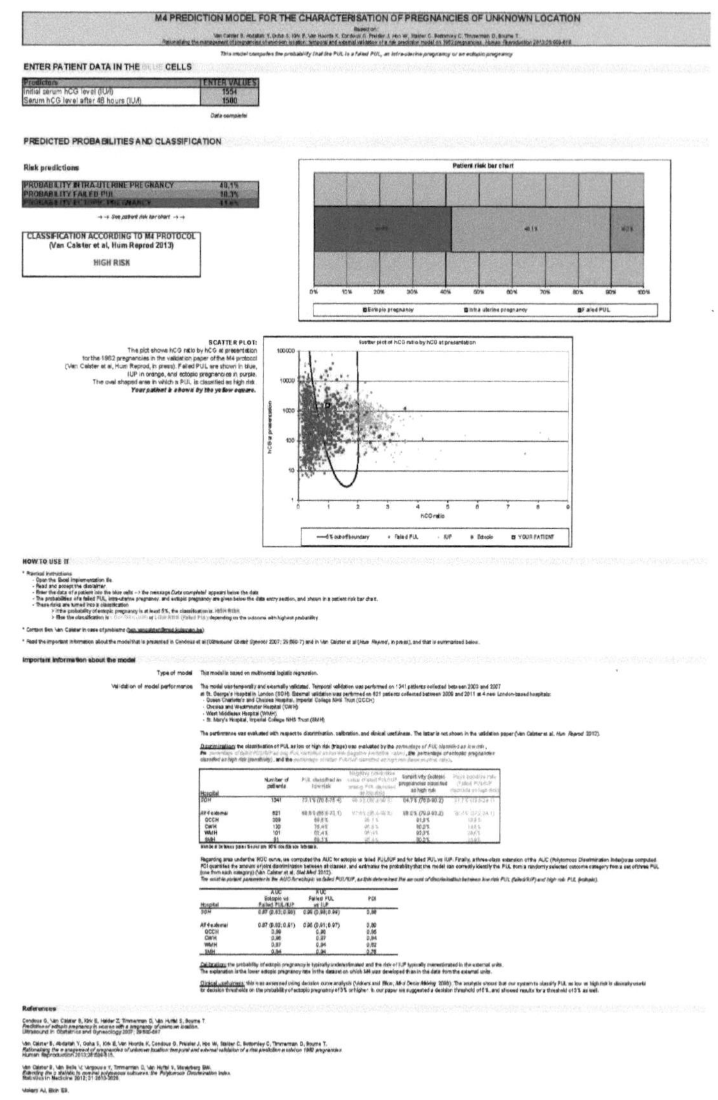

Appendix 4: Algorithm for triage and management of pregnancies with indeterminate location using the M4 model [77]

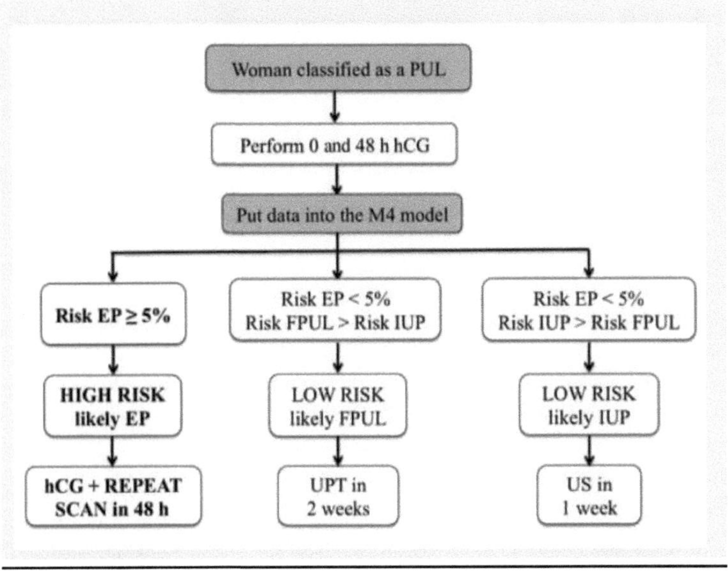

Appendix 5:

Data collection form

1) **Identité de la patiente**

   - Nom   :
   - Prénom   :
   - Numéro du dossier :   /
   - Age   :
   - Adresse   :
   - Profession :

2) **Etat civil**

   - Célibataire   ☐

   - Mariée   ☐

   - Veuve   ☐

   - Divorcé   ☐

3) **ATCDs**

   *Médicaux : Tuberculose   oui   ☐   non   ☐
   IST   oui   ☐   non   ☐

   Autres : ....

   *Chirurgicaux :   Chirurgie abdomino- pelvienne   oui   ☐   non   ☐

   Si oui à préciser :..

   Voie d'abord : Laparotomie   ☐   cœlioscopie   ☐

   *Gynécologiques :

   - Ménarche :
   - Régularité du Cycle :
   - Durée du cycle :
   - DDR :
   - Dyspareunie : Oui   ☐   Non   ☐
   - Dysménorrhée :   Oui   Non
   - Plastie tubaire : Oui   Non
   - Endométriose :   Oui   Non
   - Infertilité :   Oui   Non
        Si oui durée :......................... Ans

- **GEU :**

Si oui traitement :   médical   ☐

                        Chirurgical   ☐   : Laparotomie ☐ cœlioscopie   ☐

                                       Conservateur ☐ n conservateur   ☐

- **IGH :**
  - Si oui traitement : Médical   ☐
  -                 Chirurgical ☐   par cœlioscopie ☐ laparotomie   ☐

4) **Obstétriques :**

- Gestité :
- Parité :
- Avortements :   IVG ☐ ou Spontané ☐

                            Médical ☐ Chirurgical ☐

- Accouchement :   VB ☐
  -              CS ☐

5) **Autres FDR / HDV :**

- Tabac :   oui ☐ non ☐
  - Si oui _____ PA ☐

- Inducteur de l'ovulation : oui ☐ non ☐
- IAC :   Oui   Non
- FIV/ICSI :   Oui   Non

- Contraception :   oui   Non   Si oui, préciser : DIU ☐ micro progestatif ☐ autres ....

6) **Examen clinique :**

> Interrogatoire:

- Durée de l'aménorrhée : ....jours
- Douleurs pelviennes spontanées : oui   non
- Métrorragies : oui   non
- Signes sympathiques de la grossesse :   Nausée   ☐

                                       Vomissement   ☐

                Autres :

➢ Inspection :

- Etat général :
- Pâleur :
- Etat de conscience :

➢ Examen physique :

- Général :   *TA :

                        *FC :

                        *T :

                        *Etat abdominal :   ASED   ☐

                                        Sensibilité ou défense   ☐

                                            Si oui siège :

- Gynécologiques :
            Spéculum :   * MTR   oui ☐   non ☐
                          * Col fermé   oui ☐   non ☐

            TV : *Utérus de taille normale ☐   augmentée   ☐
                  *Masse annexielle   oui ☐   non ☐
                  * Douleur CDS   oui ☐   non ☐

7) Examens para cliniques :

➢ Biologique :   *   dosage β-HCG initial :
                        *   dosage β-HCG dans 48h :

                        * NFS : Hb :   g/dl   Plq :.............../mm^3

                            TP :   TCA :

                        *Autres

➢ Echographie :

Epaisseur de l'endomètre :

Annexes :

Epanchement : oui   non

Si oui : abondance

Autres :...

8) Durée d'hospitalisation :..........jours
9) Nombre d'échographies avant d'atteindre le diagnostic final :............................
10) Nombre de dosages de β-HCG d'atteindre le diagnostic final :...........................

11) Diagnostic final :

  - GEU :
  - GIU non évolutive :
  - GIU évolutive :
  - GIU arrêtée :

12) PEC :

Médicale : ☐

Chirurgicale :   conservateur   ☐   non conservateur   ☐

                     Laparotomie   ☐   cœlioscopie   ☐

Indication de la chirurgie :
- Echec de MTX
- Taille de la MLU>4cm :
- Epanchement de grande abondance
- syndrome fissuraire (douleurs)
- Autres :
Hémoglobine post-opératoire : ....g/dl

Abstention : ☐

Appendix 6: Protocol for managing pregnancies of undetermined location in the obstetrics and gynecology department at Ben Arous regional hospital

1. Diagnosis of pregnancies of undetermined location

Pregnancy of indeterminate location (GLI) is defined as any pregnancy that has been confirmed by a urine or blood test, but whose location cannot be determined by endovaginal ultrasound.

2. Follow-up of pregnancies of undetermined location

In our department, all women presenting with an initial diagnosis of GLI are hospitalized. They receive a series of β-HCG assays every 48 hours, at least in conjunction with endovaginal pelvic ultrasound, until a final diagnosis is made. Appropriate management is then recommended.

3. Diagnostic criteria for ectopic pregnancy

The diagnosis of ectopic pregnancy (EP) is made when :

- Stagnation of β-HCG (variation of less than 15% every 48 hours on three consecutive determinations) without appearance of ultrasound signs
- The appearance of a latero-uterine mass on ultrasound +/- effusion
- A β-HCG level >3500mUI/mL with an empty uterus
- The clinical picture of a ruptured/fissured EP

4. Management of ectopic pregnancies

4.1. Medical treatment : Methotrexate

Recommended doses are 1 mg/kg.

The most common route of administration is parenteral (IM).

Side effects: neutropenia, hepatic cytolysis, diarrhea. These effects are

Usually rapidly reversible, but require pre-therapeutic assessment.

The pre-therapeutic assessment includes :

- a complete blood count (CBC)

- a liver check-up

- and renal function

Monitoring medical treatment :

It must be rigorous: Clinical + Biological + Ultrasound

- Clinical monitoring: clinical signs to look for: pain of recent exacerbation, metrorrhagia. Physical examination: look for recent onset of tenderness.
- Biological monitoring

Quantitative measurement of ß-HCG on D0, D4 and D7, then weekly until complete negativation.

The following table summarizes medical treatment planning with MTX for GEU.

J0	Quantitative determination of ß-HCG, GS, Rhesus, RAI, CBC, Platelets, PT, APTT, Creatininemia, AST, ALT Pre-anaesthesia consultation MTX 1 mg/kg IM single dose	
J4	Quantitative ß-HCG assay Endovaginal ultrasound check-up	D4: ß-HCG level must be < 150% of initial level If > 150% and patient asymptomatic: 2nd dose of MTX*. If > 150% and clinical or ultrasound worsening: failure of medical treatment and referral to Surgery
J7	Quantitative ß-HCG assay Endovaginal ultrasound check-up	D7: HCG level < 85% of initial level

		Continue weekly ß-HCG monitoring until negativation If >85% and patient asymptomatic: 2nd dose of MTX If > 85% and clinical or ultrasound worsening: failure of medical treatment and referral to Surgery

<u>Indications for medical treatment :</u>

Medical treatment is authorized as first-line treatment only after assessment of a severity score. It is reserved for young and/or slightly progressive EPs. Sometimes, this treatment is proposed to avoid difficult laparoscopy (obesity, anesthetic risk, women who have undergone multiple operations or have multiple adhesions), or in certain particular forms of EP (after in vitro fertilization, interstitial or angular EP). Medical treatment is indicated as a second-line therapy, i.e. after failure of conservative surgical treatment (e.g. HCG levels remaining high after 48 hours of salpingotomy). In this case, an injection of methotrexate can eliminate the residual trophoblast.

4.2 Surgical treatment

Surgical treatment can be either :
- Radical: Laparoscopic salpingectomy or, more rarely, laparotomy
- Conservative: Laparoscopic salpingotomy or, more rarely, laparotomy

Post-operative monitoring of the decrease in plasma βHCG levels is essential following any conservative treatment.
Plasma β-HCG is routinely measured at 48 hours:

- If less than 15% of the initial level: therapeutic success, so no further dosage is required.
- If greater than 35% of initial rate: therapeutic failure, in the absence of clinical manifestations, additional medical treatment with methotrexate is considered
- Between 15 and 35%, the evolution is rather favorable, but requires weekly monitoring of plasma βHCG until complete negativation.

<u>*Indications for surgical treatment :*</u>

Laparotomy is indicated in cases of :

- Tubal rupture with cataclysmic hemorrhage and peritoneal flooding

- Severe shock states

- Extreme obesity

- Contraindications to laparoscopy

-Insufficient technical resources.

Elsewhere, laparoscopy is the standard approach:

4.2.1. INDICATION FOR CONSERVATIVE TREATMENT: SALPINGOTOMY :

Should always be preferred, especially if there is a desire to become pregnant. If a contralateral tube is pathological, conservative treatment should also be considered.

4.2.2. INDICATION FOR RADICAL TREATMENT: SALPINGECTOMY

- No desire for subsequent pregnancy,

- Dilapidated uterus, obvious anatomical lesions indicating a high risk of recurrence of EP

. Uncontrollable tubal hemorrhage

- Homolateral recurrence of an EP

. History of tubal plasty homolateral to EP

4.3. Therapeutic abstention

Therapeutic abstention may be proposed provided that :

-the patient is asymptomatic and can be easily monitored

Plasma β-HCG level<100 IU /ml and decrease at 48-hour intervals,

-Absence of hemoperitoneum.

TITLE	**Model M4 and HCG ratio: performance in predicting the outcome of pregnancies of unknown location**

Abstract

Introduction: Pregnancy of unknown location (PUL) presents a diagnostic and management challenge. Several biomarkers have been proposed to stratify the risk of PUL, among which the most used are serum progesterone levels, HCG ratio, and mathematical models M4 and M6. The aim of this study was to evaluate the performance of model M4 and HCG ratio in stratifying the risk of pregnancies of unknown location.

Methods: This was a single-center, retrospective, descriptive, and analytical study conducted over a period of 6 years and 4 months from January 1, 2017, to April 30, 2023, involving 384 cases of pregnancies of unknown location recorded at the Department of Obstetrics and Gynecology at the Regional Hospital of Ben Arous.

Results: We collected 384 cases of PUL. The mean age of our patients was 32.8 years. The main risk factors for ectopic pregnancy (EP) presented by our patients were: history of EP (11.3%), history of tubal surgery (4%), and history of infertility (6%). The HCG ratio had the highest sensitivity (Se) (84.6%) and negative predictive value (NPV) (99.1%) for the group of non-evolving intrauterine pregnancies (IUP) or failed PUL (HCG ratio <0.87). The highest specificity (Sp) (91.4%) and positive predictive value (PPV) (80.6%) were seen in the evolving IUP group. For the diagnosis of EP (HCG ratio between 0.87 and 1.66), the performance parameters of the HCG ratio were as follows: Se (79.3%), Sp (84.5%), PPV (76.8%), and NPV (86.4%). We established new cutoffs for the HCG ratio: a ratio between 0.77 and 1.63 had a Se of 96% with an NPV of 95.6% in predicting the risk of EP. Model M4 showed modest results in predicting the outcome of PUL using the 5% threshold (Se at 59%, Sp at 41.7%, PPV at 40.2%, and NPV at 88.7%). In our population, a threshold of 11% for model M4 provided the best compromise between Se and NPV (Se at 81%, Sp at 77%, PPV at 65%, and NPV at 90%). We developed a new predictive score for EP in patients presenting with PUL, incorporating the three statistically significant variables: an HCG ratio between 0.78 and 1.63 (OR: 3.848), initial ß-HCG >1000 IU/L (OR: 1.975), and endometrial thickness <10 mm (OR: 1.279). This score showed promising performance in predicting the risk of PUL: sensitivity of 91%, specificity of 93%, PPV of 95%, and NPV of 94%. In terms of healthcare costs, we demonstrated that the use of HCG ratio and Model M4 would lead to significant savings, particularly in the low-risk group of women.

Conclusion: The prevalence of PUL continues to rise, and its management entails high social and healthcare costs. A diagnostic strategy tailored according to risk stratification methods represents an interesting alternative for both the patient and the practitioner, as well as for the healthcare system.

<table>
<tr><td>Keywor ds</td><td>Ectopic pregnancy, Missed abortion, Mathematical model, HCG ratio, Prognosis</td></tr>
</table>

<table>
<tr><td>TITLE</td><td>

M4 model and HCG ratio: performance in predicting the outcome of pregnancies of undetermined location

</td></tr>
</table>

Summary

Introduction: Pregnancy of undetermined location (GLI) poses a diagnostic and management problem. Several biomarkers have been proposed to stratify the evolutive risk of GLI, the most widely used of which are serum progesterone, the HCG ratio and the M4 and M6 mathematical models. The aim of this study was to evaluate the performance of the M4 model and the HCG ratio in risk stratification of pregnancies with indeterminate location.

Methods: This was a mono-centric, retrospective, descriptive and analytical study conducted over a period of 6 years and 4 months, from January 1, 2017 to April 30, 2023, on 384 cases of pregnancies with undetermined location recorded in the gynecology and obstetrics department at Ben Arous regional hospital.

Results: We collected 384 cases of GLI. The mean age of our patients was 32.8 years. The main risk factors for ectopic pregnancy (EP) presented by our patients were: Previous ectopic pregnancy (11.3%), previous tubal plasty (4%) and previous infertility (6%). The HCG ratio had the best sensitivity (Se) (84.6%) and negative predictive value (VPN) (99.1%) for the group of non-progressive intrauterine pregnancies (UIP) or failed GLI (HCG ratio <0.87). The highest Sp (91.4%) and PPV (80.6%) were seen in the progressive GIU group. For the diagnosis of EP (HCG ratio between 0.87 and 1.66), the performance parameters of the HCG ratio were as follows: Se (79.3%), Sp (84.5%), PPV (76.8%) and NPV (86.4%). We established new cut-offs for the HCG ratio: a ratio between 0.77 and 1.63 had a Se of 96% with a VPN of 95.6% in predicting the risk of EP. The M4 model showed modest results in predicting the final outcome of GLI using the 5% threshold (Se at 59%, Sp at 41.7%, PPV at 40.2% and NPV at 88.7%). In our population, a threshold at 11% of the M4 model associated the best compromise between Se and VPN (Se at 81%, Sp at 77%, VPP at 65% and VPN at 90%). We developed a new score predictive of EP in patients presenting for GLI, including as variables the three statistically significant parameters: HCG ratio between 0.78 and 1.63 (OR: 3.848), initial ß-HCG >1000 IU/L (OR: 1.975) and endometrial thickness < 10 mm (OR: 1.279). This score had a promising performance in predicting the risk of GLI: sensitivity of 91%, specificity of 93%, PPV of 95% and NPV of 94%. In terms of healthcare costs, we showed that the use of the HCG ratio and the M4 Model would result in significant savings, particularly in the low-risk group.

Conclusion: The prevalence of GLI continues to rise. Its management generates high health and social costs. An adapted diagnostic strategy based on risk stratification represents an interesting alternative for patients, practitioners and the healthcare system alike.

Key words	*Ectopic pregnancy, Terminated pregnancy, Mathematical model, HCG ratio, Prognosis*

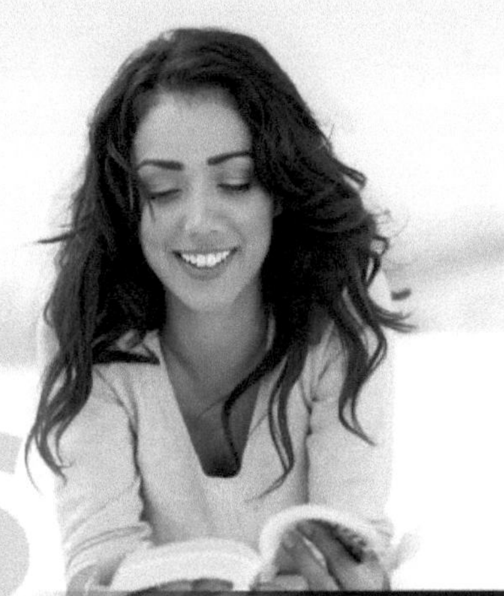

Buy your books fast and straightforward online - at one of world's fastest growing online book stores! Environmentally sound due to Print-on-Demand technologies.

Buy your books online at
www.morebooks.shop

Kaufen Sie Ihre Bücher schnell und unkompliziert online – auf einer der am schnellsten wachsenden Buchhandelsplattformen weltweit! Dank Print-On-Demand umwelt- und ressourcenschonend produziert.

Bücher schneller online kaufen
www.morebooks.shop

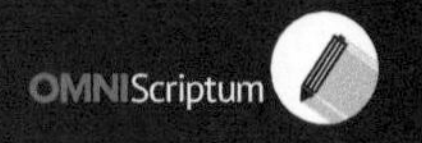

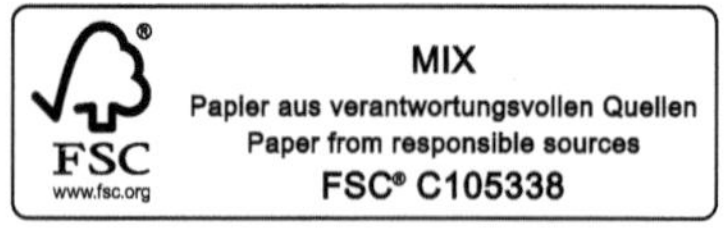

Printed by Books on Demand GmbH, Norderstedt / Germany